Clinics in Human Lactation

Breastfeeding the Late Preterm Infant
Improving Care and Outcomes

Marsha Walker, RN, IBCLC

HALEPUBLISHING

1712 N. Forest St. • Amarillo, Texas 79106 • © Copyright 2009 All rights reserved.

Clinics in Human Lactation

Breastfeeding the Late Preterm Infant

Marsha Walker, RN, IBCLC

© Copyright 2009
Hale Publishing, L.P.
1712 N. Forest St.
Amarillo, TX   79106-7017
806-376-9900
800-378-1317
www.iBreastfeeding.com
www.hale-publishing.com

Library of Congress Control Number: 2009921412
ISBN-13: 978-0-9815257-7-8

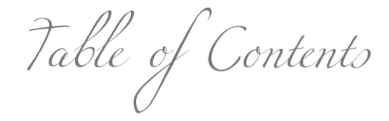

Table of Contents

SECTION 1 :: WHO IS THE LATE PRETERM INFANT?

A Population at Risk.. 5

Contributors to Late Preterm Birth.. 7

Maternal Obesity... 8

Cesarean Birth... 8

Importance of the Last Six Weeks 9

Neurological System 9

Why Human Milk is Important for Late Preterm Infants.. 12

Cardiopulmonary System 13

Thermoregulation.. 13

Energy Metabolism and Hypoglycemia... 14

Jaundice and Hyperbilirubinemia 14

Birth Interventions 15

Maternal Milk Supply 17

SECTION 2 :: BREASTFEEDING MANAGEMENT GUIDELINES WITHIN THE PHYSIOLOGICAL CONTEXT OF THE LATE PRETERM INFANT

Feeding Skills 19

Hypothermia.. 21

Hypoglycemia 23

Respiratory Instability 26

Hypotonia and Immature Feeding Skills...29

Latch Assistance 29

Supplementation 37

Use of Bottles and Artificial Nipples 40

Hyperbilirubinemia...46

Immature Self Regulation...48

Initiating and Maintaining Maternal Milk Supply 51

Fitting the Flange 51

Putting It All Together...52

Feeding Plans Following Discharge..55

CONCLUSION 57

REFERENCES...59

GLOSSARY..73

INDEX 77

AUTHOR BIOGRAPHY 81

Section One

WHO IS THE LATE PRETERM INFANT?

*A*s a clinician, how many times do you work with the frantic mother of a 36 or 38-week old baby? While medical professionals may say "He's just a little small" or "She's just a little early," these phrases actually describe a population of infants who masquerade as large, healthy, and functional, while disguising their vulnerability to a host of medical and developmental problems. These infants are not just smaller versions of a full-term baby, but are born during a period of rapid development and maturation of multiple organ and body systems. An abrupt halt to this in-utero maturation process can alter the eventual growth and development of the infant, as many systems and organs have critical windows of time where certain events need to happen for a normal outcome. Even though late preterm infants may be born healthy, they remain at a much higher risk for a host of conditions that can compromise both breastfeeding and the infant's health.

During the 1980s, babies born after 34 weeks of gestation began receiving the label "near term," the implication being that these babies were almost term and could thus be treated as such. But clinicians eventually realized that these babies posed specific challenges, even when assured that they were "fine." If a baby reached 34 weeks of gestation, it was considered a major milestone. A baby born after that time would survive and interventions to prolong the pregnancy were not necessary. Over time, 34 completed weeks of gestation came to be regarded as just about term, with 34-40 week infants combined with regard to morbidity and mortality (Raju, 2008), as well as clinical management. However, a growing body of research and clinical experience is finding that preterm birth, by even just 1 week, raises the risk for neonatal morbidity and mortality (Kramer et al., 2000; Raju et al., 2006; Wang et al., 2004).

This problem is unlikely to go away soon. The rate of premature birth in the U.S. increased almost 35 percent between 1981 and 2005, rising from 9.4 to 12.7 percent of all births (Figure 1).

Figure 1. Percentage of Preterm Births in the United States

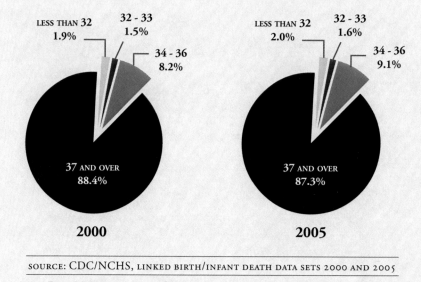

SOURCE: CDC/NCHS, LINKED BIRTH/INFANT DEATH DATA SETS 2000 AND 2005

From: MacDorman MF, Mathews TJ. NCHS Data Brief. Recent Trends in Infant
Mortality in the United States. Number 9, October 2008.

The fastest growing portion of preterm births is that of babies born between 34 0/7 and 36 6/7 weeks. This group represented 72% of the preterm births in 2005 (Figure 2) (Hamilton et al., 2007).

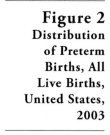

Figure 2
Distribution
of Preterm
Births, All
Live Births,
United States,
2003

From March of
Dimes, 2006

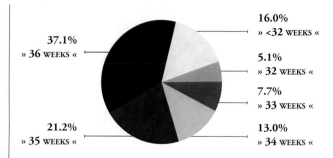

There are over 500,000 preterm births annually in the U.S. (birth prior to 37 completed weeks of gestation), 350,000 of which are late preterm. There are another 700,000 births each year that occur between 37 and 38 weeks gestation. These infants are called early term infants. Table 1 shows the nomenclature of prematurity (Hankins et al., 2006).

Table 1. Nomenclature Of Prematurity

Weeks of Gestation	Prematurity Nomenclature
<34 weeks	Preterm
34 0/7 to 36 6/7 weeks	Late Preterm
37 0/7 to 38 6/7 weeks	Early Term
39 0/7 to 41 6/7 weeks	Term
42+ weeks	Post Term

Between 1992 and 2002, the most common gestational age of singleton babies born in the United States dropped an entire week, from 40 to 39 weeks (Davidoff et al., 2006). Babies born between 37 weeks and 39 weeks are not exempt from the problems of prematurity. For example, these babies experience a 2 to 4-fold risk of complications, such as respiratory distress, NICU admission, sepsis, or hospitalization for more than 5 days (Tita et al., 2008).

Infants born at 37 and 38 weeks gestation remain at significantly increased risk for severe respiratory distress syndrome (RDS) (Bakr & Abbas, 2006). Respiratory issues are more common in late preterm infants because the pulmonary system is one of the last fetal organ systems to mature. Fetal lungs are filled with fluid that must be cleared in order for adequate gas exchange to occur after birth. In late gestation and as labor progresses, the production of lung fluid decreases and transporters in the lung that increase lung fluid clearance are induced, so that lung fluid can be cleared rapidly. Synthesis of surfactant and antioxidant enzymes also increases towards the end of the pregnancy to prepare the lungs for air breathing.

Hormonal and physiological changes associated with labor are necessary for lung maturation in neonates. These changes may not occur in infants delivered by elective Cesarean sections because of pulmonary immaturity and the lack of the beneficial effects of normal labor on the newborn. The beneficial effects of labor include reduction in lung water, enhanced catecholamine levels, secretion of surfactant stores into the alveolar space, and increased levels of pulmonary vasodilating substances.

Maternal factors can contribute to the increased incidence of sepsis or infection. Chorioamnionitis and premature rupture of the membranes may contribute not only to the etiology of preterm labor, but may also be implicated in the higher incidence of infection seen in late preterm infants (Hauth 2006). Insulin dependent diabetes also delays fetal lung development.

This shift in gestational age at birth and the associated complications of physiologically immature infants have resulted in the creation of new initiatives to improve provider and consumer awareness of this vulnerable population and to develop resources for clinicians to appropriately care for these infants. Health agencies and professional associations, such as the Association for Women's Health, Obstetric and Neonatal Nurses (AWHONN) (Askin et al., 2008) and the March of Dimes, are working on this issue.

AWHONN launched the Late Preterm Infant Initiative in 2005 as a multi-year endeavor to address the special needs of infants born between 34 and 36 completed weeks of gestation. Goals include increasing healthcare provider and consumer awareness of the risks associated with late preterm birth and ensuring evidence-based educational resources are available for nurses and healthcare providers to provide appropriate assessment and care for these vulnerable newborns. New professional resources were released in 2007, including the Late Preterm (Near-Term) Infant Assessment Guide and Optimizing Health for the Late Preterm Infant Presentation Package. AWHONN began a national multi-year research-based practice project in late 2007.

The goal of the March of Dimes Prematurity Campaign, launched in 2003, is to reduce the U.S. preterm birth rate by 15 percent. The expanded campaign is expected to address three critical areas:

1. Accelerated funding for basic research in the United States and globally and translation of the findings into practices that will benefit women of childbearing age.

2. Expansion of direct services to NICU families to provide them with information in English and Spanish about what to expect in the NICU, a glossary of common medical terminology and conditions, and tested suggestions about how to parent in a NICU.

3. The creation of community intervention programs, such as March of Dimes Healthy Babies are Worth the Wait®, which focus attention on the challenges posed by late preterm deliveries.

In July 2005, a National Institutes of Health panel recommended that this group of babies be referred to as late preterm rather than near term to better convey their greater vulnerabilities and need for closer monitoring and follow-up. The panel's opinion was that "near term" can mislead parents and clinicians into thinking that these babies are almost term and can be treated similar to term infants (Raju et al., 2006). Redefining this population of infants helps change expectations of parents and clinicians of how these babies behave and how better to anticipate care based on their unique vulnerabilities. It is hoped that better understanding of their needs and susceptibilities will reduce the problems to which they are prone. This panel also stated that gestational age should be rounded off to the nearest completed week, not to the following week. For example, an infant born on the 4th day of the 35th week (35 weeks and 4/7 days) would be considered to be a gestational age of 35 weeks, not 36 weeks.

The Federal government is concerned about the increasing rates of preterm birth. In December 2006, the United States Congress passed the PREEMIE ACT (P.L. 109-450), mandating an expansion of research, better provider education and training, and a Surgeon General's conference to address the growing epidemic of preterm births. This law was designed to improve the treatment and health of premature babies and create programs to support the emotional and informational needs of their families. By reducing the number of babies who are born below normal birth weight, this legislation will help reduce healthcare costs for states, Medicaid, and other insurers. The law authorized a Surgeon General's conference at which scientific and clinical experts from the public and private sectors sat down together to formulate a national action agenda designed to speed development of prevention strategies for preterm labor and delivery.

A POPULATION AT RISK

Late preterm infants are at an increased risk for airway instability, apnea, bradycardia, excessive sleepiness, large weight loss, dehydration, feeding difficulties, weak sucking, jaundice, hypoglycemia, hypothermia, immature self regulation, respiratory distress, sepsis, prolonged artificial milk supplementation, hospital re-admission, and breastfeeding failure during the neonatal period (Adamkin, 2006; Engle et al., 2007). The younger the baby is, the higher the risk. Some late preterm infants may take weeks to acquire competent breastfeeding skills, during which time the mother's milk supply is at risk unless regular milk expression is initiated to compensate until the infant can demonstrate adequate milk transfer. If the mother is not producing sufficient milk for infant growth, infant formula supplementation may be necessary until the milk production matches infant needs. Some mothers may also have other risk factors for insufficient milk which compound this problem (preterm delivery itself, cesarean delivery, overweight or obesity, endocrine problems, delayed lactogenesis II, insufficient pumping).

Late preterm infants, especially breastfed ones, are 2.2 times more likely to be readmitted to the hospital, especially for jaundice and infection (Tomashek et al., 2006). Wang et al. (2004) analyzed the clinical outcomes of 90 late preterm infants compared with 95 full-term infants. The analysis found significantly more medical problems and increased hospital costs for babies born between 35 and 37 weeks of gestation (Table 2). The analysis also found that late preterm infants incurred $1596 more costs than term infants.

---

[1]*http://www.marchofdimes.com/prematurity/?link=28219Title*
[2]*http://www.marchofdimes.com/aboutus/29975_29987.asp*

TABLE 2. Comparison Of Adverse Outcomes Between Late Preterm And Term Infants

Problem	Outcome Late Preterm Infant	Outcome Term Infant
Temperature Instability	10%	0%
Hypoglycemia	15.6%	5.3%
Intravenous Infusions	26.7%	5.3%
Respiratory Distress	28.9%	4.2%
Clinically Jaundiced	54.4%	37.9%
Apnea and Bradycardia	4.4%	0%
Sepsis Evaluation	36.7%	12.6%
Delayed Discharge Due To Poor Feeding	76%	28.6%

Early intervention services are increased for late preterm infants. One study found that the mean cost per child for babies born between 32 and 36 weeks was $1578 for early intervention compared to $725 for babies born at term (Clements et al., 2007).

For infants born earlier than 38 weeks, Shapiro-Mendoza et al. (2008) found that the newborn morbidity (illness) rate doubled. This risk increased when an infant was exposed to maternal hypertensive disorders of pregnancy (Table 3). Infants born at 34 weeks had 20 times the risk for morbidity compared to infants born at 40 weeks of gestation. Each week closer to 40 weeks gestation decreased the risk for morbidity - infants born at 35 weeks of gestation had 10 times the risk and infants born at 36 weeks of gestation had 5 times the risk.

Table 3. Morbidity Rates At Various Gestational Ages

Gestational Age	Morbidity Rate
38-41 weeks	2.5%-3.3%
37 weeks	5.9%
34 weeks	51.7%

Late preterm newborns have significantly higher mortality rates. Each weekly increase in gestational age is associated with a decreasing risk of death. Infants born at 37 and 38 weeks of gestation have an increase in mortality rates compared with babies born at 40 weeks.

Late preterm infants have twice the risk for sudden infant death syndrome. There were 1.4 cases per 1000 at 33-36 weeks of gestation compared with 0.7 per 1000 at >37 weeks of gestation (Kramer et al., 2000; Malloy & Freeman, 2000).

CONTRIBUTORS TO LATE PRETERM BIRTH

Numerous factors are thought to contribute to the increasing numbers of late preterm births (Table 4) (Raju et al., 2006; Engle & Kominiarek, 2008).

Table 4. Contributors To Late Preterm Birth

Late preterm births are due to increases in:
Advanced Maternal Age
Multiple Births
Medically Indicated Deliveries
Women With Chronic Diseases Becoming Pregnant
Medical Surveillance And Interventions
Maternal Obesity
Cesarean Births
Inductions And/Or Cesareans Without Medical Indication
Inaccurate Estimation Of Gestational Age During Elective Deliveries
Physician And/Or Maternal Request Or Convenience
Aggressive Management Of Hospital Staffing And Bed Turnover
Perception That Cesarean Delivery Is Easier Or Less Stressful
Changes In Medical Thresholds For Cesarean Birth

Late preterm births are due to increases in:
Belief That The Last Weeks Of Pregnancy Are Not Important
Physician Liability Concerns
Media Influence
Infertility Treatments/Invitro Fertilization

Adapted from Declercq et al, 2002; Bettes et al, 2007; Raju et al., 2006; Engle & Kominiarek, 2008.

MATERNAL OBESITY

Approximately 24.5% of women between the ages of 20 and 44 years are overweight (BMI 25.0-29.9 kg/m2); 23.0% of the women in this age group are obese (BMI >/= 30.0 kg/m2) (Vahratian, 2008). While obesity itself does not cause preterm birth, it increases the maternal medical problems that often lead to preterm deliveries, such as diabetes and hypertension. Maternal obesity and fetal macrosomia cause difficulties in estimating gestational age by ultrasound, which can lead clinicians to mistake a large fetus for a mature fetus.

CESAREAN BIRTH

The cesarean birth rate climbed to 30.3% of births in 2005 (Martin et al., 2007). The increase in the preterm birth rate, especially for late preterm births, occurred primarily among cesarean section deliveries (Bettegowda et al., 2008). There is growing concern that some of these late preterm cesarean births may be due to non-medically indicated reasons, such as convenience and patient preference or request. It has been estimated that 2.5% of cesarean births are prompted by maternal request (NIH, 2006). Others estimate that 3-18% of cesarean deliveries are elective or occur without clear medical indications (Menacker et al., 2006; Fuchs & Wagner, 2006). Both physicians and mothers may say that a planned cesarean helps them plan their schedules. Some women ask for a cesarean section because they are worried about the pain of a vaginal delivery. Wiklund et al. (2007) conducted a prospective cohort study of 357 healthy primiparas from two different groups, cesarean section on maternal request and controls planning a vaginal delivery. Mothers requesting a cesarean delivery more often reported anxiety about lack of support during labor, concerns over loss of control, and worries over fetal injury/death with a vaginal delivery. Mothers with planned cesareans were breastfeeding to a lesser extent three months after birth.

Inductions occur in 22.3% of all labors (Martin et al., 2007), two-thirds of which are elective. Because there are so many elective inductions, it takes only a small shift in clinical thresholds to opt for a cesarean delivery, greatly increasing the number of cesarean deliveries performed.

Obstetricians have noted an increased number of patients inquiring about planned cesarean delivery. Many of these physicians believe that women have the right to a cesarean delivery upon request (Bettes et al., 2007).

Iatrogenic preterm birth can be the outcome of a relaxed attitude about obstetrical interventions and women who are not fully informed about the risks of late preterm birth.

Forgotten in this departure from what nature has intended is the fact that babies mature at different rates. While they may be "safely" delivered prior to their due date, size is not an indication of maturity. Many babies need the full 40 weeks, or even a little longer, before they are sufficiently mature and ready for life outside the womb

IMPORTANCE OF THE LAST SIX WEEKS

Even though some preterm babies may look like full-term babies, late preterm infants are physiologically, metabolically, and neurologically immature and have limited compensatory mechanisms to adjust to the extrauterine environment. The last six weeks of gestation are an important period of growth and development for the fetus. During this time, subcutaneous tissue and brown fat are laid down, glycogen stores in the liver increase, antibodies are passed from the mother to the fetus through the placenta, and fetal muscle tone increases as the uterine environment becomes more restricted due to fetal growth. While all of the organ systems have formed, their final maturation occurs during the last stage of pregnancy, preparing the infant to live without the assistance of the placenta.

NEUROLOGICAL SYSTEM

At birth, the brain mass of 34-35 week late preterm infants is approximately 60% that of term infants, myelinization is markedly underdeveloped, and neuronal connections and synaptic junctions are not fully developed (Figure 3). As the billions of nerve cells (neurons) are formed in the brain over the course of 40 weeks gestation, there are a number of critical events that occur during this development, one of which is myelination. Myelin is a fatty substance that coats the axons (branches of the nerve cell), acts as an electrical insulator, and is vital to information flow along the neuron. Myelin's most important function is to speed the transmission of electrical signals, which is accomplished by the flow of ions (dissolved salts like sodium, calcium, potassium, and chloride). However, nerve

Figure 3. Striking difference between the brain of a 36 week infant and one who has reached 40 weeks

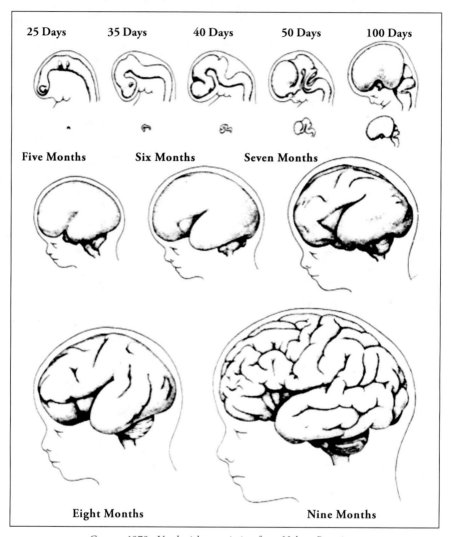

Cowan, 1979. Used with permission from Nelson Prentiss.

cells are leaky and as electrical signals speed along the length of an axon, some of the ions leak out, reducing the efficiency of the transmission. Myelination prevents this from happening by laying down a sealing coat of material that keeps ions from leaking. Such leakage can reduce the transmission of impulses all along a nerve fiber. Myelination occurs at different times in different regions of the brain. It starts in the nerve fibers of the spinal cord at 5 months of gestation, but does not begin in the brain until the last prenatal month (Eliot, 1999).

At the end of 36 weeks of gestation, the brain weight of a premature infant is about 80% the size of a term infant's brain weight (Kinney, 2006), affecting such functions as arousal, sleep-wake behavior, and the coordination of feeding with breathing. The immature brainstem adversely impacts upper airway and lung volume control, laryngeal reflexes, and the chemical control of breathing and sleep mechanisms. Ten percent of these infants experience significant apnea of prematurity (Darnall et al., 2006).

The brain of a late preterm infant is not simply a smaller version of a term infant's brain. These last weeks represent a critical window in brain development where interruption of the normal environment alters the maturational trajectory of the structure and function of the brain. If an infant is born early, the brain must complete its maturation process outside of the prenatal habitat of brain-nourishing nutrients and protection of the womb. This alters how the brain develops.

In general, children born prematurely have more problems in motor/neurologic function, visuomotor integrative skills, IQ, academic achievement, language, executive function, and attention-deficit hyperactivity disorder/behavioral issues than do their 40 week counterparts (Aylward, 2005). Volume deficiencies (smaller amounts of brain matter) in several areas of the brain can lead to behavioral and cognitive deficits when these children reach school age (Peterson et al., 2003). The degree of these abnormalities is inversely associated with measures of intelligence (Peterson et al., 2000).

Sullivan and Margaret (2003) found significant differences in total, fine, and gross motor performance, and visual-motor integration at 4 years of age between term and preterm infants. Scores for the preterm groups decreased with increasing morbidity. At 4 years of age, mild motor delay was found in all preterm groups. Children with mild motor delay had lower academic achievement scores and higher rates of school service use (special education interventions) at 8 years of age. Many children born as late preterm infants require more special education services once they reach school age.

Chyi et al. (2008) showed that late preterm infants had lower reading scores than full-term infants in kindergarten to first grade. Teacher evaluations of math skills from kindergarten to first grade and reading skills from kindergarten to fifth grade were lower for late preterm infants. Special education participation was higher for late preterm infants in early grades.

The periventricular area (the area around the spaces in the brain called ventricles) contains nerve fibers that carry messages from the brain to the body's muscles. Periventricular leukomalacia (PVL), while more commonly seen in earlier preterm infants, occurs in significant numbers of late preterm babies as well (Kinney, 2006). PVL is characterized by the death of the white matter of the brain due to softening of the brain tissue. PVL is caused by intraventicular hemorrhage, a lack of oxygen or blood flow to the periventricular area of the brain and/or bacterial infection in the mother or infant that triggers a cytokine response in the brain, resulting in the death or loss of brain tissue. This type of brain lesion injures premyelinating oligodendrocytes (cells that form and maintain the myelin sheath), resulting in an overall delay in the myelination of the brain. These cells are also vulnerable to reactive oxygen species (free radicals) that lead to further white matter damage (Kinney, 2006).

WHY HUMAN MILK IS IMPORTANT FOR LATE PRETERM INFANTS

Human milk for preterm babies of any gestational age is vital to the optimal development of a brain that has been challenged by an early birth. Breastmilk is a rich source of components designed specifically to promote brain myelinization and increased development of brain synapses, such as sialic acid-containing oligosaccharides. Higher brain ganglioside and glycoprotein sialic acid concentrations in infants fed human milk lead to enhanced developmental outcomes compared to infants fed formula (Wang et al., 2003). Human milk oligosaccharides are an important source of sialic acid, which is an integral part of the plasma membranes of nerve cells and dendrites in the brain. Formula-fed babies receive only 20% of the sialic acid that a breastfed baby receives, and formula-fed babies are not able to synthesize the difference.

Human milk's principal carbohydrate is lactose (galactose + glucose). The presence of abundant amounts of galactose is thought to help ensure an adequate supply of galactocerebrosides that are needed for myelinization. Infants fed formulas with no lactose, such as soy formula or cow's milk based formula that has had the lactose removed, consume a diet that is lacking in brain growth nutrients.

Provision of human milk is crucial to infants born preterm as these babies have a lower antioxidant capacity. This may provide a partial explanation of why they are so vulnerable to diseases and conditions associated with oxidative stress, such as necrotizing enterocolitis, chronic lung disease, retinopathy of prematurity, periventricular leukomalacia, and intraventricular hemorrhage. Breastmilk is much higher in antioxidant capacity than infant formula and helps neutralize oxidative stress in young babies (Ezaki et al., 2008).

Vohr et al. (2006) looked at younger preterm infants and found that for every 10 ml/kg per day increase in breastmilk ingestion, the Mental Development Index increased by 0.53 points, the Psychomotor Development Index increased by 0.63 points, the Behavior Rating Scale percentile score increased by 0.82 points, and the likelihood of rehospitalization decreased by 6%. Infants receiving the most breastmilk enjoyed a 5 point elevation in IQ, or conversely, infants fed no breastmilk experienced a 5 point IQ deficit.

With their diminished muscle tone, late preterm infants are more prone to positional apnea due to airway obstruction. Their immature autonomic system may demonstrate exaggerated responses to stressful stimuli with rapid or lower heart rates, abnormal breathing, skin mottling, frequent startling, regurgitation, or simply shutting down. Their ability to self regulate may be limited. They may appear to be irritable, difficult to console, and/or not very responsive to their parents' overtures.

CARDIOPULMONARY SYSTEM

Late preterm infants are at a greater risk for lung morbidities because they are born during a period of time when alveoli are maturing, surfactant levels are increasing, and the lungs are changing from fluid secretion organs to fluid absorption organs. Birth prior to lung maturation delays amniotic fluid clearance, reduces maintenance of alveolar expansion, and decreases lung perfusion. It places these infants at risk for respiratory distress syndrome, transient tachypnea, bradycardia, and respiratory failure. It also predisposes them to persistent pulmonary hypertension. Birth by cesarean section in the absence of labor further exacerbates these conditions.

Apnea occurs more frequently as the late preterm infant may be less sensitive to higher levels of carbon dioxide and may experience decreased upper airway dilator muscle tone (Engle et al., 2007). They may also be at increased risk for centrally mediated apnea because their central nervous systems are developmentally immature, with fewer sulci and gyri in the brain and less myelin. Late preterm infants also have twice the risk for sudden infant death syndrome (Malloy & Freeman, 2000).

THERMOREGULATION

Temperature instability is a common problem in late preterm infants. Brown fat stores, maturation of the processes needed to mobilize these stores, and hormones involved in brown fat metabolism do not peak until term (Stephenson et al., 2001; Symonds et al., 2003). Full term infants enjoy a full complement of glycogen stores in the liver and possess the ability to oxidize subcutaneous brown fat which provides energy reserves during the period directly after birth. Late preterm infants possess less subcutaneous fat for insulation, their skin is a poor barrier to evaporative heat loss, and they cannot generate heat from brown adipose tissue as well as a full-term infant can. Preterm infants lose heat more readily than a term infant because of their larger ratio of surface area to body mass. When exposed to cold stress, they must rely on immature mechanisms of increasing metabolism for heat, including the use of glucose and glycogen stores. The relative lack of glycogen stores culminates in a quick depletion of glucose and the development of hypoglycemia. Hypothermia can worsen pre-existent respiratory distress and hypoglycemia.

ENERGY METABOLISM AND HYPOGLYCEMIA

At birth, the newborn's glucose concentration is about 80% of maternal glucose, but levels decline rapidly to one-third of the maternal concentration (40 to 60 mg/dl) by 30 to 90 minutes following delivery. In the late preterm infant, this concentration may be as low as 30 to 40 mg/dl (Ward Platt & Deshpande, 2005). Late preterm infants are at a higher risk for hypoglycemia due to their diminished glycogen stores and immature hepatic energy pathways. Their counter-regulatory efforts are less efficient as they have difficulty generating glucose until their metabolic pathways can compensate. Late preterm infants have difficulty developing an alternate fuel source for the brain as their ketogenic response is often diminished. Many lack adequate fat to contribute to glucogenesis and may be unable to compensate due to inadequate intake of breastmilk. They can also be affected by other conditions, such as sepsis and cold stress, which contribute to hypoglycemia.

Hyperinsulinism may be encountered in infants of diabetic mothers and in babies whose mothers are obese and insulin-resistant. A cascade of conditions may occur whereby the infant of a diabetic mother grows large and has a cesarean section, leading to a late preterm infant who appears big and heavy, but is physiologically immature. Given the increase in overweight and obesity in the U.S., the incidence of gestational diabetes has risen. The outcome results in more macrosomic infants who run the risk of becoming late preterm babies, with hyperinsulinism and the resulting hypoglycemia (Heiskanen et al. 2006; King, 2006).

JAUNDICE AND HYPERBILIRUBINEMIA

Late preterm infants' delayed maturation causes them to experience a combination of factors that put them at a 7 to 13-fold increased risk for re-hospitalization for jaundice (Maisels & Kring, 1998), including slower meconium passage, decreased activity of the bilirubin-conjugating enzyme - uridine diphosphate glucuronyl transferase (UGT), and low breastmilk intake. Jaundice occurs when conditions unique to the newborn interfere with the production, conjugation, and or excretion of bilirubin. Depending on the gestational age of the infant, initial meconium passage may occur after 24 hours post birth and may be prolonged over a period of 4 to 6 days (Bekkali et al., 2008). This presents a greater opportunity for the bilirubin reservoir in meconium to re-enter the infant's circulation and contribute to continuously rising bilirubin levels that exaggerates jaundice in this population. Jaundice is the main reason late preterm infants are re-admitted to the hospital (Shapiro-Mendoza et al., 2006).

Bilirubin levels in some infants can rise high enough to cause neurologic damage if not closely monitored or if interventions are not implemented soon enough to lower extremely high levels. If bilirubin reaches very high levels in susceptible infants, it can cross the blood-brain barrier and damage specific areas of the brain. The American Academy of Pediatrics (AAP) recommends the term acute bilirubin encephalopathy be used to describe the condition where clinical signs are seen in the early weeks following birth. The term kernicterus refers to the chronic and permanent clinical outcomes of bilirubin toxicity, which can include athetoid cerebral palsy, hearing loss, paralysis of upward gaze, dental dysplasia, and possibly intellectual handicaps. Kernicterus is seen more frequently in late preterm infants (Bhutani & Johnson, 2006). Breastmilk feeding is almost universally present, with large for gestational age babies, male sex, and G6PD deficiency over-represented in late preterm infants with kernicterus (Watchko, 2006). Bilirubin peak levels generally occur around 2 to 3 days in term infants; however, peak bilirubin levels in late preterm infants typically occur around 5 to 7 days of life (Sarici et al., 2004). A baby born at 36 weeks has a 6-fold higher risk of eventually developing a total serum bilirubin level greater than 20 mg/dl compared with a full-term 40 week infant (Newman et al., 2005).

The AAP clinical management guidelines on hyperbilirubinemia categorize 35-36 week infants at high risk for hyperbilirubinemia. Infants delivered at 37-38 weeks are considered to be at moderate risk for hyperbilirubinemia, and babies delivered at 39 weeks and beyond are in the low risk category (American Academy of Pediatrics Subcommittee on Hyperbilirubinemia, 2004).

Many clinicians use a nomogram, a graph that looks at the infant's age in hours post birth and bilirubin level, to predict the likelihood of exaggerated or severe jaundice (Bhutani et al., 1999). A nomogram that may be a more appropriate alternative for use with the late preterm newborn uses nomograms for various gestational ages (Maisels & Kring, 2006).

Dehydration secondary to poor feeding and reduced milk intake exacerbates the development of high bilirubin levels, as jaundice is often accompanied by low weight gain or dehydration (Gartner & Herschel, 2001). Poor feeding can consist of a number of indicators, such as failure to latch, poor latch that does not transfer milk, weak sucking pressures, inability to sustain nutritive sucking long enough to ingest sufficient quantities of milk, and excessive sleepiness that leaves infants underfed. Climbing bilirubin levels at any gestational age signal the need for increasing breastfeeding support. An IBCLC lactation consultant should be utilized to prepare a breastfeeding plan of care.

BIRTH INTERVENTIONS

In addition to a late preterm infant's multiple systems immaturity, events and interventions during the peripartum period can also pose a challenge to breastfeeding. Mothers who experienced a cesarean delivery have reported that the pain associated with the procedure significantly interfered with their ability to breastfeed their infant during the hospital stay (Karlström et al., 2007). Postoperative pain is not limited to the immediate postpartum time frame, as women who have undergone a cesarean section may report problems with pain for as long as 4 to 8 weeks after the surgery (Schytt et al., 2005). Pain and stress are known to inhibit the milk ejection reflex (Newton & Newton, 1948), which may limit the amount of milk a baby receives at each feeding. Only small volumes of milk (1-10 ml) can be either expressed (Kent et al., 2003) or obtained by the breastfeeding infant (Ramsay et al., 2004) prior to activation of the milk ejection reflex. A late preterm infant simply may not possess the stamina to sustain sucking until the milk lets down or be too fatigued to feed once it does.

Type of anesthesia can also impact an infant's ability to feed well. Infants may experience hypotonia (low muscle tone) from the maternal use of labor medications, such as nalbuphine (Nubain). Normal muscle tone is necessary for the lips to maintain a seal on the breast, for the jaw and tongue to work in a coordinated manner, and for vacuum to be exerted to facilitate the flow of milk from the nipple/areola. Newborns should be monitored for respiratory depression, apnea, bradycardia, and arrhythmias if Nubain has been used (Food and Drug Administration, 2005).

Intrapartum fentanyl contained in epidural analgesia may also impede the establishment of breastfeeding. Jordan et al. (2005) showed that the higher the dose of fentanyl, the more likely women were to be bottle-feeding at hospital discharge. Fentanyl is sequestered in the fetus (Bader et al., 1995; Loftus et al., 1995), who has a higher concentration of unbound opioids than the mother. Fentanyl concentration further increases if the infant becomes acidotic from crying or a cesarean delivery (Helbo-Hansen, 1995). The human body functions best when blood and tissue fluids are neither too alkaline nor too acidic. An abnormally high acidity of blood and tissue fluids is called acidosis and results in chemical reactions taking place less efficiently.

Elimination half-lives (the time required for half of a quantity of a drug to be metabolized or eliminated by the body) of fentanyl are longer in neonates than adults. The half-life of fentanyl in the neonate is between 3-13 hours (Hale, 2008). It takes about 5 half-lives to eliminate or metabolize drugs from the body, implying that some infants will have been discharged prior to complete metabolism of fentanyl. The elimination of fentanyl in neonates is not always uniform and can involve transient rebounds (periodic rises), which can prolong depressant effects (Koehntop et al., 1986). Delayed clearance of fentanyl allows it to accumulate in the central nervous system, which can produce subtle behavioral changes, such as depression of feeding reflexes (Steer et al., 1992; Desprats et al., 1991). Beilin et al. (2005) demonstrated that women who were randomly assigned to receive high-dose fentanyl in their epidural reported difficulty breastfeeding more often than women who were randomly assigned to receive an intermediate fentanyl dose or no fentanyl. Neurobehavior scores were lowest in the infants of women who were randomly assigned to receive more than 150 micrograms of fentanyl. At 6 weeks postpartum, more women who were randomly assigned to high-dose epidural fentanyl were not breastfeeding compared to women who were randomly assigned to receive either an intermediate fentanyl dose or no fentanyl. Use of maternal labor medication may further compromise the late preterm infant's feeding ability.

Labor medications also increase the risk of assisted birth. For example, epidural analgesia is a risk factor for the use of vacuum extraction (O'Hana et al., 2008). Instrument assisted births pose the potential for head trauma that can affect breastfeeding. Instrumental vaginal delivery involves the use of the vacuum extractor or obstetric forceps to facilitate delivery of the fetus. It is associated with substantial risk of head injury, including hemorrhage, fractures, and, rarely, brain damage or fetal death (Doumouchtsis & Arulkumaran, 2008). Late preterm infants suffer more complications from vacuum extraction, such as scalp edema, bone fracture, and cephalhematoma, than do full-term infants (Simonson et al., 2007). Hall et al. (2002) demonstrated that vacuum extraction was a strong predictor of breastfeeding cessation by 7 to 10 days.

Fetal exposure during the third trimester to selective serotonin reuptake inhibitors (SSRIs) has also been reported to cause feeding difficulties (Nordeng & Spigset, 2005). Levinson-Castiel et al. (2006) compared the prevalence and clinical characteristics of neonatal abstinence syndrome in neonates exposed and not exposed to SSRIs in utero. One hundred and twenty term infants were studied. Sixty of these infants had prolonged in utero exposure to SSRIs, including paroxetine hydrochloride, fluoxetine, citalopram hydrobromide, sertraline hydrochloride, and venlafaxine hydrochloride. Thirty percent had neonatal abstinence syndrome; eight cases were severe. The most common symptoms were tremor, gastrointestinal problems, abnormal increase in muscle tone (hypertonicity), sleep disturbances, and high-pitched cries. Symptoms were most prominent during the first 48 hours following birth. Alterations in alertness, muscle tone, feeding, gastrointestinal distress, and neurological parameters were noted in 73 neonates exposed to anti-depressants in late pregnancy compared with 73 neonates with no exposure (Boucher et al., 2008). In-hospital clinicians working with breastfeeding mothers who have taken SSRIs during pregnancy need to be extra vigilant in regards to the infant's breastfeeding behaviors. Mothers and babies should be kept together and engage in skin-to-skin contact to help the infant modulate and regain state control.

Maternal Milk Supply

Mothers of late preterm infants may be at increased risk of delayed lactogenesis II. Lactogenesis II is the onset of copious milk production following delivery. This usually takes place between 32 and 96 hours postpartum. Delayed lactogenesis II is defined as greater than 72 hours postpartum and less than 9 g/feeding at 60 hours of age. Mothers with delayed lactogenesis II may be overweight or obese, have experienced a cesarean delivery (Dewey et al., 2003), be of advanced maternal age, have a history of infertility, have pregnancy induced hypertension, diabetes, or been treated for preterm labor (Chapman & Perez-Escamilla, 1999).

The onset of lactogenesis can be delayed between 15 and 28 hours in women with insulin dependent diabetes mellitus (Arthur et al., 1989; Hartmann & Cregan, 2001; Neubauer et al., 1993). Rasmussen and Kjolhede (2004) showed that the prolactin response to suckling was reduced in overweight and obese mothers and that this diminished response lasted up to 7 days postpartum. Maternal and fetal stress during labor and delivery are associated with impaired lactogenesis (Dewey, 2001). Preterm birth itself often compromises the initiation of lactation, delaying the onset of copious milk production (Cregan et al., 2002) and presenting a prolonged colostral phase to an infant with immature feeding skills.

Breastmilk transfer over the first 6 days of life has been shown to be less in full-term babies whose mothers experienced a cesarean delivery compared to those born vaginally (Evans et al., 2003). In a study to determine hormonal pattern release differences between vaginally and cesarean delivered mothers, Nissen et al. (1996) showed that the number of oxytocin pulses occurring during the first 10 minutes of the breastfeeding session varied between 0 and 5. The vaginally delivered mothers had significantly more pulses than the mothers delivering by cesarean section. Furthermore, the mothers who had cesarean sections lacked a significant rise in prolactin levels at 20-30 minutes after the onset of breastfeeding. These conditions may limit the amount of milk available to the infant during the early days. Late preterm infants with limited breastfeeding skills and reduced breastfeeding efficiency and whose mothers present colostrum for an extended period of time are at risk for slow or no weight gain, dehydration, and hyperbilirubinemia. Their mothers are at risk for insufficient milk production.

Section Two

BREASTFEEDING MANAGEMENT GUIDELINES WITHIN THE PHYSIOLOGICAL CONTEXT OF THE LATE PRETERM INFANT

FEEDING SKILLS

Late preterm infants are at a disadvantage in terms of feeding skills. They are born with low energy stores (both subcutaneous and brown fat). They have high energy demands, poor feeding abilities, and are sleepy, with fewer and shorter awake periods. They tire easily when feeding, have a weak suck and low tone, demonstrate an inability to sustain sucking, and may have a small mouth, with uncoordinated oral-motor movements. They are easily over-stimulated and may shut down before consuming adequate amounts of colostrum or milk. They may take only small volumes of milk during the early days in the hospital, which are often sufficient for that period of time, but exhibit feeding difficulties when higher volumes of milk intake become necessary for normal growth. While some babies may demonstrate adequate muscle tone initially, this tone may be rapidly depleted during a feeding, indicating decreased endurance. Postural stability may be immature, creating a less efficient feeding pattern. During the last weeks of pregnancy, the space within the uterus becomes more confined as the fetus grows. This results in more flexion of the extremities and increased muscle tone (Pados, 2007). Full term infants achieve muscle tone that is mature enough to maintain the airway, grasp, draw, and keep the nipple/areola in their mouth, and generate sufficient vacuum to effect milk transfer. Late preterm infants experience reduced tone in the muscles involved with feeding, which coupled with neurologic immaturity of the suck, swallow, breathe cycle results in uncoordinated and ineffective milk intake at the breast. If treated like a normal term newborn, they are at an increased risk for inadequate nourishment. They may go through the motions of feeding, but may transfer little if any milk for their efforts.

Sucking parameters vary among the gestational ages and even in infants of the same gestational age. Very preterm infants have the capacity to engage in the rudiments of breastfeeding, with attainment of full breastfeeding varying greatly, depending on their health status and the amount of access the baby has to the breast (Nyqvist, 2008). Sucking competency matures from weak sucking, a partial seal on the mother's breast, short sucking bursts, long pauses between bursts, small amounts of milk per suck, occasional swallowing, several swallows per suck and several sucks per swallow, breath holding, and short suck duration (Furman & Minich, 2006; Meier & Pugh, 1985) to coordination between sucking, swallowing, and breathing in a 1:1:1 pattern over a sustained period of time.

Effective breastfeeding depends greatly on the infant's ability to draw the maternal nipple into the oral cavity, maintain it there with about -60 mm Hg over the entire feeding, and generate enough vacuum through the action of the tongue/jaw dropping to facilitate milk flow from the breast. Intraoral vacuum also depends on an oral cavity that is sealed, i.e., the lips and facial muscles possess enough tone to initiate and maintain a seal over the nipple and areola (Wolf & Glass, 1992).

Ultrasound scans show a feeding sequence in which a space is created in the infant's mouth when the tongue/jaw drops, into which milk is delivered following the milk ejection reflex. Milk-filled ducts are drawn into the nipple as it elongates with vacuum applied by the baby. With the tongue at its most upward position, it holds the nipple in contact with the palate, but does not appear to compress any milk into the mouth. Tongue movement downward posterior to the nipple tip is followed by milk exiting the nipple. The nipple typically rests immediately anterior to the hard and soft palate junction (Jacobs et al., 2007).

Geddes et al. (2008) demonstrated that in term infants, vacuum plays a major role in removing milk from the breast, with milk flowing only when vacuum is applied. In this study, intraoral pressure was lower in younger babies. This may help to partially explain why late preterm infants encounter difficulty with sufficient milk transfer, as their ability to generate high enough vacuum levels may be compromised by their low muscle tone, rapid decrease in tone during a feeding, poor seal on the breast, and difficulty in maintaining the nipple in an optimal position.

Bromiker et al. (2006) noted poorer sucking patterns among full-term infants of insulin-managed diabetic mothers when measured while feeding on a bottle. Diabetic mothers treated with insulin had infants who averaged fewer sucking bursts and fewer sucks per 5-minute interval. Several reports have described an association between maternal diabetes and less optimal neurobehavior in the infant, especially if the diabetes was not well controlled. This suggests that infants of diabetic mothers may be less neurologically mature (Georgieff, 2006).

Rizzo et al. (1990) found that with increasing maternal serum glucose levels during the second and third trimester, the newborn infants' responses on the Brazelton Neonatal Behavioral Assessment Scale (BNBAS) were poorer. Shulte et al. (1969) described more immature electroencephalography patterns in infants of diabetic mothers compared with controls, suggesting a delayed neural maturation. Pressler et al. (1999) showed that infants of diabetic mothers had poorer motor processes and reflexes on the BNBAS.

Maternal diabetes can affect the development of the fetal and neonatal nervous system, with the result being poor neurologic outcomes in offspring, not only in the neonatal period, but also when the child reaches school age (Ornoy et al., 2001). Maternal diabetes can, therefore, have the potential to further complicate the feeding issues surrounding the late preterm infant if an already immature nervous system meets yet one more challenge to its ability to control feeding.

The creation of a breastfeeding plan of care for late preterm infants is predicated by their vulnerabilities. Breastfeeding management options for this population are often extrapolated from those used with either full-term infants or with infants less than 34 weeks of gestation, neither of which may be completely appropriate for the unique needs of the late preterm population. Not all interventions are well researched, but the clinician may find the evidence-based protocols for breastfeeding the late preterm infant in Table 5 helpful when working with this population. Breastfeeding interventions are designed to accomplish three goals: prevent adverse outcomes, establish the mother's milk supply, and assure adequate infant intake.

Hypothermia

If the baby and mother are stable immediately following birth, babies should be placed skin-to-skin on the mother's chest. In this position, they should be dried, covered with warm blankets, and have a cap placed on their head. Extended skin-to-skin contact

Table 5. Evidence-Based Hospital Breastfeeding Protocols For Late Preterm Infants

Protocol	Available from	Comments
California Perinatal Quality Care Collaborative. Care and Management of the Late Preterm Infant Toolkit: Nutrition.	*http://www.cpqcc.org/ quality_improvement/ qi_toolkits/care_and_ management_of_the_late_ preterm_infant_toolkit*	Toolkits are all inclusive packages to help facilitate improved clinical outcomes, excellent patient care and efficient resource allocation.
The Academy of Breastfeeding Medicine. Protocol #10: Breastfeeding the near-term infant (35 to 37 weeks gestation).	*www.bfmed.org/ace-files/ protocol/near_term.pdf*	

keeps the infant warm, reduces crying (Matthiesen et al., 2001), and allows for frequent breastfeeding, all of which help prevent hypoglycemia. Newborns placed skin-to-skin with mothers remain considerably warmer during the first 3 hours following birth, compared with newborns swaddled in mother's arms or receiving nursery care (Bystrova et al., 2003). Bathing the infant should be delayed for at least 2 to 3 hours to allow temperature stabilization.

Bergman et al. (2004) showed that preterm infants provided skin-to-skin care by their mothers had better physiological outcomes and stability than infants separated and cared for in closed servo-controlled incubators. They explained that the cardio-respiratory instability seen in separated infants during the first 6 hours post birth is consistent with mammalian "protest-despair" biology and with "hyper-arousal and disassociation" response patterns described in human infants. These are particular side effects of separating infants from their mothers. These separation reactions function as a defense program in the infant, with their own set of hormones, autonomic controls and somatic expressions. The "protest" response is one of intense activity, with the infant seeking to reunite with the mother. The "despair" response is a withdrawal and survival response, with decreased temperature and heart rate in the infant, mediated by a massive rise in stress hormones.

Babies interact more with their mothers and are more likely to be breastfed and to breastfeed longer if they have early skin-to-skin contact. Late preterm infants show better cardio-respiratory stability if they have early skin-to-skin contact (Moore et al., 2007). Babies should be assisted to the breast for their first feeding within an hour or so of birth. If the mother experienced a cesarean delivery, her baby should stay with her and she should be assisted to breastfeed in the recovery room. Dabrowski (2007) reported that following a cesarean delivery, infants placed in skin-to-skin contact with mothers en route to post-anesthesia recovery are often alert and attempting to breastfeed upon arrival at the recovery room. They achieve thermoregulation (normal body temperature) more rapidly than newborns placed under a radiant warmer.

Colson et al. (2003) described a strategy during the hospital stay called biological nurturing that involved holding late preterm newborn infants so that their chest, abdomen, and legs were closely flexed around a maternal body contour and unrestricted access to the breast was offered, with abundant skin-to-skin contact. Rather than leaving infants in a bassinet between feedings, mothers were encouraged to hold the infant in a biological nurturing position. The authors suggested that during the 40 weeks of a full term pregnancy, mothers cannot put their infants down, so physiologically the infant could continue to be incubated or gestated in the mothers' arms during the early days following a late preterm birth. When mothers picked up on feeding cues, infants who appeared to be asleep were observed to be actively sucking at the breast. After the infant was seen to complete a suck/swallow cycle, another cycle was more easily triggered, suggesting that flow regulates suck, and that the more swallows achieved, the more sucking that followed. This study suggested that mothers assume a semi-reclining position with entire frontal aspect of the baby's body draped prone around a natural contour of the mother's body.

HYPOGLYCEMIA

While closer monitoring for hypoglycemia is warranted for late preterm infants, breastfeeding is an important part of any hypoglycemia protocol (Academy of Breastfeeding Medicine, 2006). Especially if the mother is diabetic, breastfeeding attempts should occur:

- Within 1 hour after birth
- Once every hour for the next 3 to 4 hours
- Every 2 to 3 hours until 12 hours of age
- At least 8 times each 24 hours during the hospital stay

Frequent breastfeeding is important for late preterm infants who lack stamina and demonstrate inefficient feeding skills. However, unless swallowing takes place and is documented during these feeding sessions, late preterm infants may actually receive little colostrum, exacerbating hypoglycemia. A sample feeding plan (Table 6) for the mother to follow for her late preterm infant will help reduce the risk of hypoglycemia and serve as a general guide for breastfeeding in the early days. Skills necessary for her to accomplish this plan should be taught to her and should include how to latch the infant correctly at the breast, how to know when the infant is behaviorally available to feed based on infant feeding cues, how to tell if the infant is swallowing colostrum/milk, how to do alternate massage, how to hand express colostrum into a spoon, and how to feed it to her infant.

Table 6. Sample Breastfeeding Plan For Mothers

The Plan	Details
Feed your baby frequently	• Within 1 hour after birth • Once every hour for the next 3 to 4 hours • Every 2 to 3 hours until 12 hours of age • At least 8 times each 24 hours during the hospital stay
Place baby skin-to-skin on your chest	
Watch for rapid eye movements under the eyelids (baby will wake easily)	
Move baby to breast when baby shows feeding cues	• Sucking movements of the mouth and tongue • Rapid eye movements under the eyelids • Hand-to-mouth movements • Body movements • Small sounds

The Plan	Details
Make sure you know how to tell when baby is swallowing	• Baby's jaw drops and holds for a second • You hear a "ca" sound • You feel a drawing action on the areola and see it move towards baby's mouth • You hear baby swallow • You feel the swallow when you place a finger on baby's throat • Your nurse hears the swallow when a stethoscope is placed on baby's throat
Use alternate massage if baby doesn't swallow after every 1 to 3 sucks	Massage and squeeze the breast each time baby stops between sucks. This helps get more colostrum into her and keeps her sucking longer
If your baby does not swallow when at the breast, hand express colostrum into a teaspoon (Figure 4) and spoon feed 2 teaspoons to your baby using the above guidelines	

In between feedings, mothers can be instructed to keep their baby skin-to-skin and avoid separations. Christensson et al. (1992) noted a 10mg/dl drop in blood glucose levels when term infants were removed from their mother and placed in a bassinet.

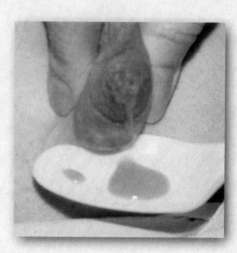

Figure 4
Hand Expressing
Colostrum Into
A Spoon

From
The Breastfeeding Atlas,
4th Ed., Wilson-Clay
& Hoover, 2008.
Used with permission.

RESPIRATORY INSTABILITY

Careful positioning for breastfeeding is necessary to avoid apnea, bradycardia, or desaturation, especially for younger babies with decreased muscle tone. They are more prone to positional apnea due to airway obstruction and should not be fed in positions that cause excessive flexion of the neck or trunk. The traditional cradle hold is one of the positions to avoid, as babies can become so flexed that full rib cage expansion is impeded and the risk of airway collapse is increased. Some infants may prefer slight extension in their neck to keep their airway open. Cross cradle (Figure 5) or clutch (Figure 6) are positions of choice (Meier et al., 2007). The cross cradle position has the mother supporting the baby with the arm and hand opposite of the breast being suckled. The palm of the hand supports the shoulders; the thumb and index finger encompass the base of the head and are placed just below the ears. The rest of the mother's arm supports the trunk of the infant in slight flexion. The clutch position places the baby to the side of the breast being suckled. This can be modified to allow for gradations, from a baby lying almost flat to being elevated into a "V" shape, depending on how best the baby feeds. When utilizing the clutch position, care should be taken to assure that the breast does not rest on the baby's chest (Figure 7 and Figure 8), further impeding breathing and rib cage expansion. The cross cradle and clutch positions prevent the baby from engaging in extreme flexion of the trunk and neck.

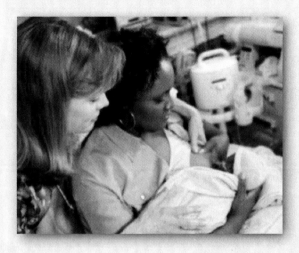

Figure 5
Cross cradle
position
assures straight
alignment of
head and trunk

From
Medela Inc. Copyright
© 2008 Medela. All
Rights Reserved.

Figure 6
Clutch position
with mother's
hand at the
base of the head
around the
neck. Hands
are correctly
positioned off
of the occiput
(back part of
the head)

From
Medela Inc. Copyright
© 2008 Medela. All
Rights Reserved.

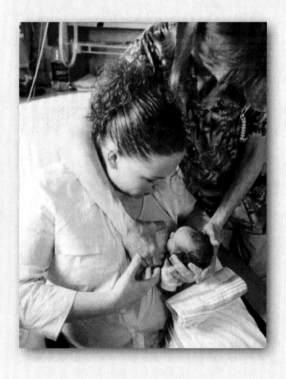

Preterm infants lack postural control in their necks (cervical area) and may have difficulty maintaining stability during feedings. Some infants feed better when swaddled, as their arms are brought to midline and their entire body is stabilized. A mother can be advised to use breastfeeding positions where her hand can encircle the occipital region (back) of the baby's head. This head support maintains the head alignment, compensates for the lack of postural control in the neck and weak neck musculature, and helps prevent the infant from slipping off the breast.

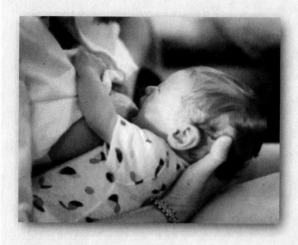

Figure 7

Infant in clutch position, with weight of large breast pressing on chest. Mother's hand should be moved lower, off of the occiput

Photo courtesy of Marsha Walker. Used with permission.

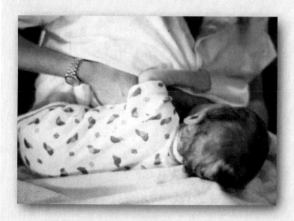

Figure 8

Infant repositioned to side-lying clutch position removing weight from chest

Photo courtesy of Marsha Walker. Used with permission.

HYPOTONIA AND IMMATURE FEEDING SKILLS

Some babies may be able to effectively latch, suck, and swallow colostrum, especially with jaw support. Others will tire quickly, be unable to sustain nutritive sucking, or lack the strength to draw the nipple/areola into the mouth and generate the -60 mm Hg (Geddes et al., 2008) of pressure necessary to maintain it there. Late preterm infants demonstrate a wide range of variations in sucking patterns, sucking intensity, and the frequency and duration of pauses between sucking bursts. Nyqvist et al. (2001) used surface electromyography in a study of sucking patterns in 26 infants aged 32-37 weeks. The time actually spent engaged in sucking ranged between 10% and 60% of a feeding, while mouthing movements other than sucking ranged from 2-35% of the feeding and pauses ranged from 12-67% of a feeding.

LATCH ASSISTANCE

If babies have poor muscle tone, mothers may find that using the Dancer hand position (Figure 9) helps stabilize the jaw so the baby does not keep slipping off the nipple or does not bite or clench the jaws to keep from sliding off the breast (Danner & Cerutti, 1984).

Some infants may need assistance in opening their mouth wide enough to draw in the entire nipple plus part of the areola, as they do not exhibit spontaneous mouth opening or do not open their mouth wide enough. Eliciting the rooting reflex may help, as mouth opening is a central component of this reflex. For some infants, mothers can be instructed to gently exert downward pressure on the chin to open the mouth and turn out the lower lip (Wolf & Glass, 1992) (Figure 10).

If the infant latches, but smacking sounds can be heard, this may signal that the infant's tongue is losing contact with the nipple/areola as the jaw drops down too far. Sublingual pressure may be useful to keep the tongue in contact with the breast. Sublingual pressure is done when the mother slips her index finger directly behind and under the tip of the chin where the tongue attaches, limiting the downward movement of the jaw so that suction is not broken each time the jaw drops.

An engorged areola or areolar edema may complicate latch attempts by presenting large inflexible tissue that the infant may not be able to surround with his mouth. It may appear that the nipple is flat, but rather it may be enveloped by edematous areolar tissue. Placing a vacuum pump on swollen tissue to pull out the nipple may exacerbate

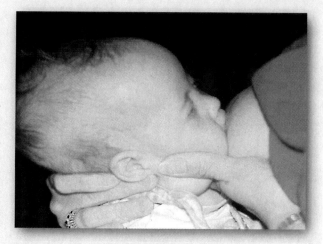

Figure 9
Dancer hand
position

From
Wilson-Clay & Hoover,
2002. Used with
permission.

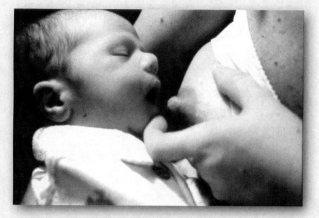

Figure 10
Assisting the
infant's mouth
to open wide
for latch on

Photo courtesy of
Marsha Walker. Used
with permission.

the problem. If the areola is engorged, areolar compression (Miller & Riordan, 2004) or reverse pressure softening (Cotterman, 2004) can be utilized to displace fluid in the areola for an easier latch. This involves the mother pressing her fingers around the areola to make indentations or pits that serve to expose the nipple (Figure 11).

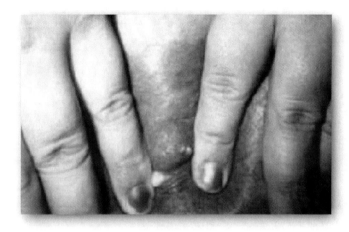

Figure 11

Mother pressing edematous areola to form pits around the nipple

From Cotterman, K.J. (2004). Reprinted by permission of Sage Publications.

If flat nipples are compromising latch, consider using a modified syringe to evert the nipple (Kesaree et al., 1993). A 10 ml syringe is modified by cutting ¼" above where the needle attaches, removing the plunger, and inserting it into the cut end. Prior to a feeding, the smooth end is placed over the nipple and the mother pulls back gently on the plunger for 30 seconds (Figure 12). Commercial devices used to evert flat nipples include the Evert-It Nipple Enhancer™ (Maternal Concepts, Elmwood, WI) and the LatchAssist™ (Lansinoh Laboratories, Alexandria, VA)

Figure 12
Steps to modify syringe to evert nipples

From Kesaree et al., 1993. Reprinted with permission of Sage Publications.

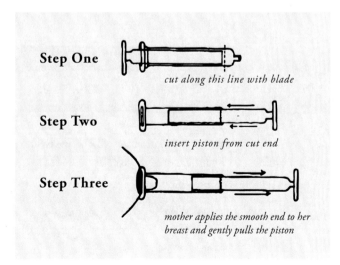

Step One

cut along this line with blade

Step Two

insert piston from cut end

Step Three

mother applies the smooth end to her breast and gently pulls the piston

Alternate massage/breast compressions (Figure 13) may be helpful to sustain sucking and increase the amount of colostrum or milk transferred at a feeding. The mother massages and compresses the breast each time the baby pauses between sucking bursts, doing so on each breast at each feeding. This helps improve the pressure gradient between the breast and the mouth, reducing the effort necessary to withdraw milk. Mothers should make sure that all quadrants of each breast are massaged and compressed to prevent milk stasis and a down regulation of milk production from a lack of adequate drainage.

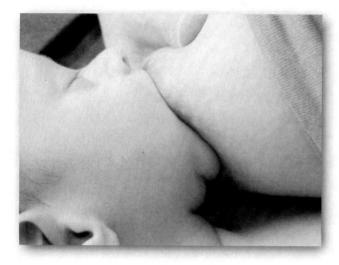

Figure 13

Breast compressions alternating with sucking bursts

From *Dr. Jack Newman's Visual Guide to Breastfeeding*, Kernerman & Newman, 2007. Used with permission.

The clinician may use a milk-filled dropper as an incentive to assist the non-latching infant to attach to the breast or to assist the infant who is engaging in rapid side-to-side head movements to latch. Some infants who are overly hungry demonstrate a deteriorating behavioral pattern at the breast, with rapid head movements or arching away from the breast. As the mother guides the baby forward to the breast, touching the midline of the upper lip with the tip of a milk-filled dropper will stop the head movements and orient the baby to the breast (Figure 14). As the baby latches, a drop or two of milk can be placed on the tongue to encourage a swallow followed by a nutritive suck (Figure 15).

Once the infant can reliably latch to the breast and transfer milk, mothers can help strengthen the infant's suck by using a nipple tug technique. As long as the mother's nipples are not sore, she can gently tug back on the nipple (or pull the baby slightly away from

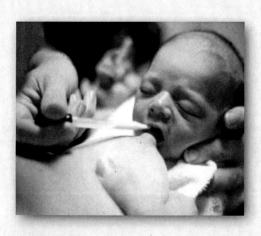

Figure 14
Dropper
assisted latch
stops rapid side-
to-side head
movements

Photo courtesy of
Marsha Walker. Used
with permission.

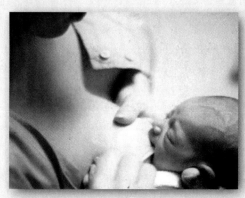

Figure 15
A milk
incentive causes
the infant to
swallow and
follow with a
nutritive suck

Photo courtesy of
Marsha Walker. Used
with permission.

her) while the infant is latched, causing him to draw the nipple/areola farther back into his mouth to maintain the latch. This technique will often cause the baby to engage in nutritive sucking after a pause and can be used to help sustain sucking during feedings.

If other latch assist techniques fail to improve the infant's latch, use of an ultrathin silicone nipple shield may be helpful to initiate latch and compensate for weak sucking, as preterm infants often repeatedly lose contact with the nipple, slipping off the breast and necessitating multiple attempts to re-latch. Careful shield use has resulted in very young preterm infants consuming more milk at feedings (Meier et al., 2000). Select the size (16 mm, 20 mm, or 24 mm) that best fits the baby's mouth (a 24 mm size may be too big for younger infants). The mother should moisten the shield with warm water and turn it almost inside out when applying it to the nipple (Figure 16).

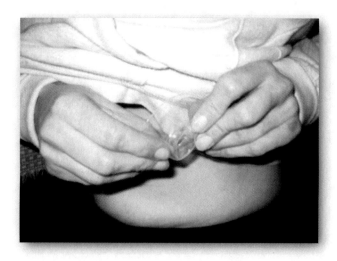

Figure 16
Applying the nipple shield

Photo courtesy of Marsha Walker. Used with permission.

This helps the shield stay in place better and places the nipple as far into the nipple tunnel as possible. The mother can hand express some colostrum/milk into the shield tunnel to make it immediately available to any amount of sucking. Once the nipple has been drawn into the shield, a vacuum in the semi-rigid teat assures that the nipple stays elongated and lowers the workload on the baby of having to constantly draw the nipple/areola back into the mouth. Mothers can also place a few drops of colostrum or milk on the tip of the shield to encourage latch on. The baby should be checked to make sure the lips and gums completely cover the shield tunnel (Figure 17) and that he is not just gumming the tip of the shield. Use of thin silicone shields has not resulted in compromised prolactin levels (Chertok et al., 2006).

Figure 17
Shield-assisted latch. The infant's mouth is wide open and completely covering the nipple tunnel and part of the areola

From Wilson-Clay & Hoover, 2002. Used with permission.

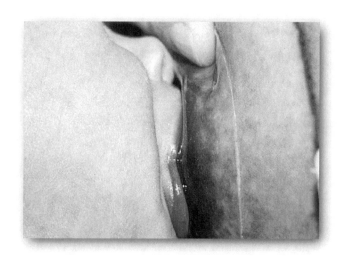

Mothers may need to check that all areas of each breast are adequately drained while using a shield. Any areas of milk stasis should be massaged and compressed. Shields can be washed in hot soapy water, rinsed, and air dried between feedings. If the infant cannot transfer sufficient milk with the shield in place and is unable to latch without it, a tube from a tube feeding device can be placed under or on top of the shield to deliver pumped milk supplements. As the infant's sucking improves, mothers generally try latching without the shield or remove it partway through a feeding, as they gradually wean the infant from the shield.

ASSESSING FEEDINGS AT THE BREAST

Infant competence in breastfeeding occurs along a continuum of oral motor behaviors. Immature or disorganized sucking patterns can limit milk intake in infants with gestational ages below term. Nyqvist (2008) demonstrated that even very preterm infants (gestational ages between 26 and 31 weeks) showed emerging competence in breastfeeding behaviors over time as they met milestones in breastfeeding capacity. These infants were able to ingest sufficient daily volumes of breastmilk at a low maturational level primarily due to the extended presence of the mother in the NICU and the abundant practice opportunities these infants enjoyed at the breast. The Preterm Infant Breastfeeding Behavior Scale (PIBBS) (Table 7) provides a useful tool to observe the emerging competence in oral motor behavior during breastfeeding over time (Nyqvist et al., 1996). Even if an infant's sucking pattern is not fully mature, he still may be capable of intake of milk volumes sufficient for adequate growth at that time. Much of the early success of the late preterm infant being capable of feeding at the breast depends on abundant practice opportunities. Keeping the infant in extended skin-to-skin care in the early days facilitates the mother's milk production and earlier attainment of breastfeeding (Hake-Brooks & Anderson, 2008; Hurst et al, 1997). Use of the PIBBS gives the clinician a mechanism to track the emerging breastfeeding competencies of the infant. The items are not scored as the tool is intended for observational and tracking purposes over the continuum of skill acquisition. It can provide anticipatory guidance to the mother regarding what she can expect over time regarding the specific breastfeeding behaviors indicative of movement to a mature feeding status. Meeting of these milestones is often an incentive to persevere with breastfeeding over the potentially many weeks it takes to achieve breastfeeding competence.

Table 7. The Preterm Infant Breastfeeding Behavior Scale (PIBBS)

Scale items	Level of competence
Rooting	• Did not root • Showed some rooting behavior (mouth opening, tongue extension, hand-to-mouth/face movements, and head turning)
Areolar grasp (How much of the areola is inside the baby's mouth)	• None, the mouth only touched the nipple • Part of the nipple • The whole nipple, not the areola • The nipple and some of the areola
Sucking	• Not licking • Licking and tasting but no sucking • Single sucks, occasional short sucking bursts (2-9 sucks) • Repeated (2 or more consecutive) short sucking bursts, occasional long bursts (10 sucks or more before a pause) • Repeated long sucking bursts
Longest sucking bursts	• Maximum number of consecutive sucks
Swallowing	• Swallowing not noticed • Occasional swallowing noticed
Latched to the breast	• Did not latch on at all; not felt by the mother • Latched on for <1 minute • Latched on for 1-15 minutes

From Nyqvist et al., 1996.

SUPPLEMENTATION

If the infant cannot obtain adequate colostrum or milk directly from the breast with the use of frequent cue-based feeds, alternate massage, milk incentives at the breast, or with the shield in place, supplementation may be required. The best supplement is expressed colostrum/milk or banked human milk if available. Feeding volumes of 5 to 10 ml every 2 to 3 hours on the first day, 10-20 ml on day two, and 20-30 ml on day three are suggested (Stellwagen et al., 2007). Mothers can hand express colostrum into a spoon and spoon feed this to the infant (Hoover, 1998). One teaspoon equals 5 ml. If a pump is used to express colostrum, small amounts may cling to the sides of the collection container leaving little for actual use. Pumping into a small container, such as an Ameda diaphragm or the Medela colostrum collection container, that has been placed between the valve and the collection bottle of either an Ameda or Medela breast pump may yield a greater quantity of usable colostrum (Figure 18).

Diabetic mothers may wish to express colostrum prenatally, freeze it, and bring it to the hospital with them should their infant need supplementation during the hospital stay (Cox, 2006). Infants of diabetic mothers are at higher risk for hypoglycemia. A

Figure 18. **Placement of Ameda diaphragm between valve and collection container**

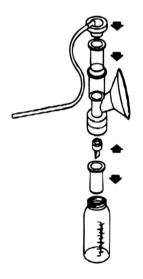
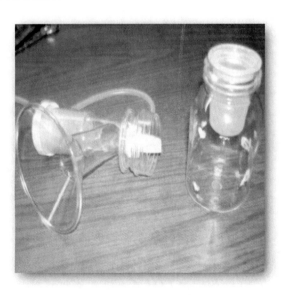

From Ameda Breastfeeding Products. Used with permission.

ready supply of colostrum eliminates the need to supplement with infant formula should the mother have difficulty expressing colostrum in the hospital. If supplementation is necessary, providing human milk rather than cow's milk-based formula avoids the possible sensitization of an infant who may be genetically predisposed to develop diabetes (Vaarala et al., 1999).

Diabetic mothers can begin to hand express colostrum at 34 weeks if there are no contraindications. Each breast is expressed for 3 to 5 minutes once a day. If cramping occurs while expressing, prenatal colostrum expression should be stopped. Mothers have the option of using a 1 or 3 ml syringe to draw up drops of colostrum, or they can express directly into a small container. These containers should be labeled and frozen, then brought to the hospital.

If a baby cannot gain appropriate weight with adequate volumes of breastmilk, more calorie dense hindmilk can be used as a supplement, the breastmilk can be fortified, or infant formula can be used temporarily until the baby is fully established at the breast. Use of a hydrolyzed formula will reduce the risk of sensitizing a susceptible infant to allergies (Greer et al., 2008) or diabetes and may simultaneously help lower bilirubin levels (Gourley et al., 2005).

There are a number of different ways to supplement a breastfed infant (Figure 19) (Stellwagen et al, 2007).

Supplementation should be done at the breast if at all possible. A 5 French feeding tube can be attached to a 10 ml syringe for supplementation at the breast. The tubing can be taped to the breast, placed under or over a shield, or held in place by a helper. Similar devices can be created from a length of butterfly tubing (with the needle removed) attached to a 20 ml or 30 ml syringe (Edgehouse & Radzyminski, 1990). Small boluses can be used if needed to help the baby initiate and sustain sucking, as flow regulates suck. Commercial tube feeding systems are available for short or longer term supplementation.

The flow rate can be adjusted with any of the commercial supplementer devices to either augment flow or avoid overwhelming a baby with low endurance. If the infant is holding his breath, looking distressed, sputtering, or coughing, the flow needs to be slowed so that a comfortable ratio of sucking to swallowing is seen and the baby inhibits breathing only when swallowing (Wolf & Glass, 2008). Mothers may wish to use the clutch position to maintain good head control. Care must be taken to assure a deep latch so the infant is not simply sucking on the tubing like a straw (Guoth-Gumberger, 2006).

Figure 19. Tube, cup, and finger feeding methods of supplementing the breastfed infant

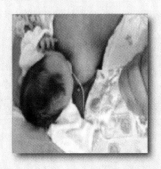

5- or 10-mL syringe containing expressed human milk and/or formula can be attached to a 5 Fr feeding tube, the end of which should be inserted along the infant's palate after she/he has latched properly onto the breast. The syringe should be slowly pushed when the infant sucks.

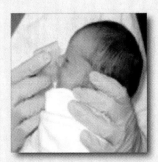

During "cup feeding" the infant is supported in a slightly upright position. A small cup containing supplement is placed at the bottom lip to stimulate mouth opening. The cup is then tilted so that the baby can slowly sip.

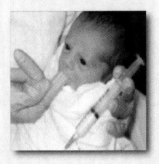

For "finger feeding" supplement is drawn into a 5- or 1-mL syringe, which is then attached to a 5-Fr feeding tube. The end of the tube should be supported by a gloved finger when introduced into the infant's mouth. As the infant sucks on the finger, the syringe plunger can be slowly pushed.

Cup feeding allows participation of the masseter and temporalis muscles, similar to how they function in breastfeeding (Gomes et al., 2006). The masseter muscle is involved in chewing, biting, swallowing, and speech. It contributes to accurate movements of the mandible (lower jaw). The temporalis muscle is responsible for raising the mandible. Howard et al. (1999) found that during cup feeding, full-term infants maintained physiologic stability and appropriate oxygen saturation. The researchers found that this method of supplementation was both effective and time efficient. Cup feeding has also been shown to be a safe and easily learned technique for supplementing preterm infants (Marinelli et al., 2001). Howard et al. (2003) reported that cup feeding had a beneficial effect on breastfeeding outcomes in a vulnerable population of mothers delivered by cesarean section when multiple supplemental feedings were required. Cup feeding led to a significantly longer duration of breastfeeding when more than two supplemental feedings were given.

USE OF BOTTLES AND ARTIFICIAL NIPPLES

Perioral muscle function differs between bottle-feeding and breastfeeding, with a weakening of masseter muscle activity in bottle-fed infants (Inoue et al., 1995). Buccinator muscles are recruited to compensate for altered tongue function during bottle-feeding. Changes in tongue function alter and weaken other muscles, such as the styloglossus and palatoglossus, used during sucking and swallowing. This change in oral muscle function may contribute to an infant experiencing difficulty in transitioning to the breast after being bottle-fed (Ferrante et al., 2006). There can be significant differences between bottle-feeding and breastfeeding in terms of swallowing and the stability of the suck-swallow-breathe cycle (Goldfield et al., 2006). Mizuno and Ueda (2006) reported that sucking pressures for nutritive and non-nutritive sucking are exactly the opposite when comparing breastfeeding and sucking on an artificial nipple. Random, frequent, and uncoordinated swallowing seen with some bottle-feeding systems can contribute to desaturation, poor intake, and a delay in breastfeeding skill acquisition.

If supplementation will be done by bottle, choice of an artificial nipple can be problematic. Nipple flow rates are not standardized; many nipples are too stiff for an infant with a weak suck; some have rapid flow rates that compromise ventilation; and none fit the anatomic shape of an infant's oral structures. The mechanics of sucking on specific artificial nipples have been sparsely studied (Fadavi et al., 1997; Goldfield et al.,

2006) and care must be taken in interpreting the results as nipple parameters (material, deflection, and extension capabilities) are changed frequently by manufacturers.

When choosing an artificial nipple for a breastfed baby, consider the following. The artificial nipple should have a soft nipple (silicone rather than latex) that can be slightly elongated and deflected upward, mimicking the shape changes of the human nipple/ areola. The human nipple is not stationary during breastfeeding and has a mean movement of 4.0 + 1.3 mm during infant sucking (Jacobs et al., 2007). If the strength required to alter the artificial nipple shape is beyond the infant's capacity, the tongue may be forced down, reinforcing an incorrect swallow pattern (Ferrante et al., 2006).

The length of the artificial nipple is also important. Jacobs et al. (2007) found on ultrasound scans that the nipple tip of the human nipple was usually not drawn into the mouth to a point where it rested directly under the junction of the hard and soft palate, but was positioned approximately 5 mm in front of this spot. The artificial nipple should not be so long that it causes the baby to gag. Shorter, softer, more mobile nipples may result in a supplementation experience that does not compromise the transition to feeding at the breast.

If a bottle is used, paced feedings are important to avoid fatigue, bradycardia, and desaturation in the baby. Paced feeding is utilized when infants are not able to coordinate respiration with sucking and swallowing (Van den Berg, 1990). Palmer (1993) recommends that the feeder regulate the number of sucks per burst and the duration of bursts and pauses by removing the nipple from the infant's mouth every 3-to-5 sucks, allowing a 3-to-5 second pause for breathing. When the bottle is removed from the infant's mouth, the nipple rests on the midpoint of the upper lip during the breathing pauses, remaining available to allow the infant to open his mouth and draw in the nipple when ready to feed (Genna et al., 2008). This helps direct control of the feeding to the infant rather than having the feeder insert the nipple. Late preterm infants of younger gestational ages (34-35 weeks) may benefit from leaving the nipple in the baby's mouth while tipping the bottle downward to stop the flow of liquid into the mouth. During the absence of flow from the nipple, the infant has time to take breaths and swallow without accumulating more milk in the oral cavity (Law-Morstatt et al., 2003).

Finger feeding is not well researched, but can be useful for short term supplementation of breastfed infants. It can be incorporated into a plan of care for establishing or transitioning an infant back to feeding at the breast. A tube feeding device can be held or taped to a feeder's finger that is held pad side up as the baby is encouraged to draw the finger into his mouth. A small bolus of milk is delivered to the infant when he sucks.

While some infants require the milk bolus as a method of suck conditioning, many infants are able to remove milk from the device on their own. This is thought to occur when the baby engages in sucking movements that mimic sucking at the breast. Finger feeding can be used prior to a feeding to prepare the infant for attempts at breastfeeding or after a breastfeeding to deliver supplemental milk if needed. A periodontal syringe (a syringe with a curved tip) may also be used to deliver supplement at the breast or as a tool for finger feeding. Table 8 summarizes the strengths and limitations of many of the devices used for supplementation or for assisting the infant to feed at the breast.

The use of a rented digital infant scale that can measure weight changes within 1 to 2 g might be appropriate post discharge when clinicians must closely watch intake or when determining the amount of supplement a particular infant needs. Mothers of preterm infants are typically quite concerned about whether their infant is getting enough milk at each feeding, whether the baby is gaining weight, and if and how much supplement the infant may need (Hurst et al., 2004). Mothers may know they have an adequate milk supply, but remain uncertain whether the infant is removing sufficient amounts of milk during feedings or needs to be supplemented (Kavanaugh et al., 1995). During the early days at home, late preterm infants may continue to breastfeed inefficiently. Pre- and post-feed weights will validate whether the infant received sufficient intake or needs to be either supplemented after each feeding or supplemented once or twice each day with expressed breastmilk or infant formula. With an infant scale, parents can track weight gain over time, reducing the need for frequent trips to the infant's primary healthcare provider for simple weight checks.

Supplementation may need to continue following discharge, sometimes until the infant reaches his due date or even for several weeks beyond. Information on supplementation should be included in a discharge feeding plan. Even when adequate breastmilk is available, infants with immature breastfeeding skills may not be able to consume all of what they require until their actual due date or longer (Hurst et al., 1999). Supplements can be gradually decreased based on a number of parameters that are unique to each infant:

- Improvement in pre- and post-feed weights when nursing directly on the breast without use of tube feeding supplementers

- Continued adequate weight gain when supplement amounts are gradually decreased

- Increasing amounts of supplement left in tube feeding devices or feeding bottles

- Maternal perception of post-feed breast fullness

Table 8. Advantages and Disadvantages of Alternative Feeding Devices

Feeding Device	Advantages	Disadvantages
Tube feeding devices	• Allow all feedings at the breast • Avoid artificial nipples and the potential for altering oral structure configurations • Reinforce correct sucking patterns • Stimulate milk production • Deliver needed nourishment • Allow flow rate to be adjusted to meet baby's needs • May assist in sustaining sucking in a weakly sucking infant by providing milk flow at the breast	• Can be awkward, messy, and take time to learn • Can be time consuming when cleaning equipment • May be used improperly if baby sucks on the tube like a straw • Make it difficult to feed away from home • Can be a problem if parts break • May be expensive for some parents
Finger feeding	• May help infant mimic correct oral conformation • Requires a wide open mouth with the tongue down, cupped, and forward. Reduces tongue tip elevation • Can be used to deliver supplement as well as prime infant for feeding at the breast	• Can be a problem if infant displays difficulty in drawing mother's nipple/areola into the mouth because baby has become accustomed to a rigid finger • Does not stimulate milk production

Table 8. Advantages and Disadvantages of Alternative Feeding Devices

Feeding Device	Advantages	Disadvantages
Syringe	• Can be used to deliver milk incentives at the breast to encourage latch • Can be used with finger feeding to supply small amounts of milk prior to going to breast for calming purposes and suck training • Delivers milk rewards for sucking attempts	• Often needs another person to deliver milk incentives at the breast • Has the potential to overwhelm the infant if milk is forcefully injected into the mouth • Is a time consuming way to feed a baby
Cup feeding	• Preserves function in muscles used to breastfeed • Is easy to learn and use avoids artificial nipples • Is a rapid way to supplement • Is safe - reducing apnea and bradycardia seen with bottle-feeding • Is a noninvasive alternative to gavage feeding	• Does not teach infant to feed at the breast • May cause the loss of significant amounts of milk if infant dribbles, making intake more difficult to quantify (Dowling et al., 2002) • Increases the risk of aspiration if milk is poured into the infant's mouth (Thorley, 1997) • Does not increase milk production

Table 8. Advantages and Disadvantages of Alternative Feeding Devices

Feeding Device	Advantages	Disadvantages
Nasogastric tube feeding in the hospital	• Assures adequate intake in infants who are unable to suck effectively, especially younger late preterm infants • Avoids artificial nipples • Is temporary	• Is invasive • Does not improve milk production
Artificial nipples	• Are a quick and easy way to supplement • May need to be considered if long term supplementation is necessary • Are helpful in certain situations when specialized artificial nipples are needed	• May cause mother to abandon breastfeeding • May overwhelm infant if nipple has a fast flow rate • May cause apnea and bradycardia during feedings • Alters oral conformation, tongue movement, and muscle function

HYPERBILIRUBINEMIA

Four preventive goals can help reduce jaundice-related complications (Stellwagen et al., 2007).

1. Optimize milk intake by feeding the infant 10 or more times each 24 hours, assuring that the baby is swallowing colostrum/milk at these feedings. Frequent feeds do not assure adequate intake unless the baby is actually swallowing during most of the feeding. Check that the baby has a deep latch, add alternate massage, and use a nipple shield if weak sucking pressure prevents good intake.

2. Promote quick meconium clearance.

3. Increase stool volume through the use of frequent colostrum feeds. If the infant cannot obtain colostrum directly from the breast, the mother can hand express colostrum into a spoon and spoon feed this to the baby frequently during the day.

4. Prevent excessive weight loss. Assure that feedings are not missed or skipped due to the presence of visitors or excessive interruptions. One feeding per shift should be observed by a nurse or lactation consultant to document that swallowing is taking place and that the mother can state when her baby is swallowing milk. The use of pre- and post-feed weights should be considered if there is significant doubt as to baby's intake at the breast.

The measurement of total serum bilirubin and transcutaneous bilirubin levels for newborns prior to discharge and the use of a nomogram is becoming a common practice in many hospitals and is recommended by the AAP (AAP Subcommittee on Hyperbilirubinemia, 2004) as a predictor of subsequent hyperbilirubinemia. These data are useful for detecting worrisome trends, identifying infants who need additional evaluation, and planning appropriate follow-up care for jaundiced newborns. Maisels and Kring (2006) have constructed bilirubin nomograms for infants 35 to 37 6/7 weeks and 38 to 39 weeks (Figure 21). An infant with rising bilirubin levels or an infant in the higher risk categories alert clinicians to the need for more intensive lactation services. Mothers will benefit from a referral to a lactation consultant upon discharge for close follow-up (Hillman, 2007). Mothers whose babies are at very high risk for jaundice can be discharged with a handheld bilirubin meter for closer monitoring over the first week of life. Late preterm infants should be seen by their primary care provider within 48 hours of discharge. It is important that mothers make this appointment prior to being discharged from the hospital and that they are reminded of the importance of keeping this appointment.

Figure 21. Bilirubin nomograms for various gestational ages

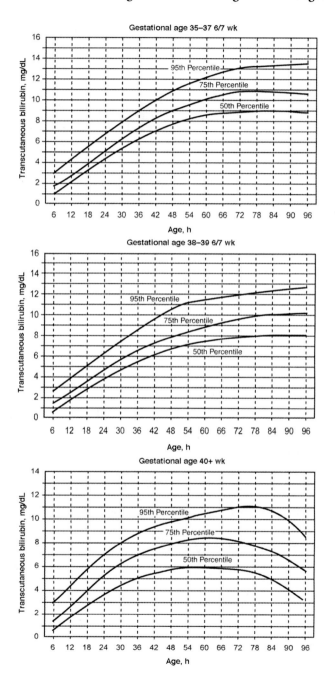

Maisels & Kring, 2006. Used with permission.

IMMATURE SELF REGULATION

More than one-third of the brain volume at term is acquired during the last 6 to 8 weeks of gestation, leaving late preterm infants at a disadvantage in responding to stimuli and regulating internal processes. Major influences on the initial pattern and ultimate duration of breastfeeding include the ability of the infant to suck efficiently, demonstrate alertness and stamina, and possess the ability to self-regulate and respond to maternal soothing behaviors (Lothian, 1995). Late preterm infants may have difficulty with self regulation as the autonomic nervous system is usually immature. This means that they may respond in a negative manner to stressful stimuli with tachycardia, bradycardia, abnormal breathing, skin mottling, frequent startling, and spitting up. Karl (2004) described behavioral breastfeeding difficulties on a continuum, from the under-aroused sleepy baby through the quiet alert state (optimal for feeding) to the over-aroused fussy, reluctant nurser. For infants unable to manage their state well enough to latch, skin-to-skin care can be initiated to modulate infant state for the under-aroused, over-aroused, or shut down infant. Handouts can be provided to parents and/or posters can be displayed in hospital labor, delivery, recovery, and postpartum rooms encouraging mothers and clinicians to keep infants skin-to-skin with their mothers (Figures 22 & 23). Parents should be aware that stroking, massaging, rocking, talking, bright lights, loud noise, and being handed off to multiple visitors may cause the baby to shut down. Infants experiencing state overload may appear to be sleeping, but may be shut down in an effort to protect themselves from excessive stimulation that raised their arousal levels beyond what they can manage. Shut down babies demonstrate tense muscle tone, furrowed eyebrows, tightly shut eyes, and a pale or flushed color. More stimulation to these babies further exacerbates the problem. Parents need to become knowledgeable regarding how best to help their baby achieve a latchable state. Only one activity at a time should be engaged in. Since alert periods are scarce, mothers should be putting the baby to the breast at these times. It is best to limit visitors during the first 2 weeks and work to minimize the dozens of interruptions that mothers experience each day during the hospital stay (Morrison et al., 2006).

Figure 22. Handout/poster encouraging mothers to keep their infants skin-to-skin during the hospital stay

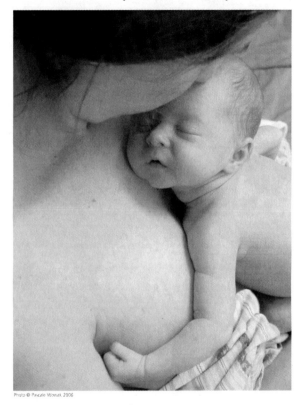

From Massachusetts Breastfeeding Coalition, www.massbfc.org. Used with permission.

Figure 23. Handout/poster encouraging skin-to-skin care beyond the hospital stay

It's my birthday,
give me a hug!

Skin-to-Skin Contact for You and Your Baby

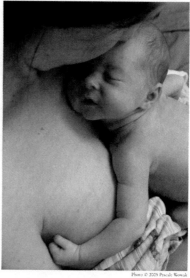

Photo © 2005 Pascale Wowak

 What's "Skin-to-Skin"?

Skin-to-skin means your baby is placed belly-down, directly on your chest, right after she is born. Your care provider dries her off, puts on a hat, and covers her with a warm blanket, and gets her settled on your chest. The first hours of snuggling skin-to-skin let you and your baby get to know each other. They also have important health benefits. If she needs to meet the pediatricians first, or if you deliver by c-section, you can unwrap her and cuddle shortly after birth. Newborns crave skin-to-skin contact, but it's sometimes overwhelming for new moms. It's ok to start slowly as you get to know your baby.

Breastfeeding

Snuggling gives you and your baby the best start for breastfeeding. Eight different research studies have shown that skin-to-skin babies breastfeed better. They also keep nursing an average of six weeks longer. The American Academy of Pediatrics recommends that all breastfeeding babies spend time skin-to-skin right after birth. Keeping your baby skin-to-skin in his first few weeks makes it easy to know when to feed him, especially if he is a little sleepy.

A Smooth Transition

Your chest is the best place for your baby to adjust to life in the outside world. Compared with babies who are swaddled or kept in a crib, skin-to-skin babies stay warmer and calmer, cry less, and have better blood sugars.

Bonding

Skin-to-skin cuddling may affect how you relate with your baby. Researchers have watched mothers and infants in the first few days after birth, and they noticed that skin-to-skin moms touch and cuddle their babies more. Even a year later, skin-to-skin moms snuggled more with their babies during a visit to their pediatrician.

Skin-to-Skin Beyond the Delivery Room

Keep cuddling skin-to-skin after you leave the hospital– your baby will stay warm and comfortable on your chest, and the benefits for bonding, soothing, and breastfeeding likely continue well after birth. Skin-to-skin can help keep your baby interested in nursing if he's sleepy. Dads can snuggle, too. Fathers and mothers who hold babies skin-to-skin help keep them calm and cozy.

About the research

Multiple studies over the past 30 years have shown the benefits of skin-to-skin contact. In all the studies described here, mothers were randomly assigned to hold their babies skin-to-skin or see them from a distance. For more information, see Anderson GC, GC. Moore, E. Hepworth, J. Bergman, N. Early skin-to-skin contact for mothers and their healthy newborn infants. [Systematic Review] *Cochrane Pregnancy and Childbirth Group Cochrane Database of Systematic Reviews.* 2, 2005.

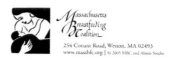

Massachusetts Breastfeeding Coalition
254 Conant Road, Weston, MA 02493
www.massbfc.org | © 2005 MBC and Alison Stuebe

Some late preterm infants (especially those of higher gestational ages) may do well with cue-based feedings, signaling to feed frequently enough to ingest adequate amounts of milk. However, not all late preterm infants will thrive using the highly flexible feeding patterns seen in full term breastfeeding infants. They may need more of a semi-structured feeding pattern as some will not be able to make up necessary volumes of milk when left to sleep for long periods of time. An infant left to sleep for 5 hours a couple of times each day may quickly fall behind and not be able to make up for their volume after so many hours of sleep (Ludwig, 2007). Use of behavioral feeding cues becomes paramount in catching the infant when he is most likely to feed well.

INITIATING AND MAINTAINING MATERNAL MILK SUPPLY

Initiation and protection of the maternal milk supply starts in the hospital. If the baby is unable to transfer colostrum, then hand expression or pumping should be started within 6 hours of delivery (Hill et al., 2001). Anecdotal reports describe some mothers as having a considerable colostrum bolus available by pump immediately following delivery. Should the baby be unable to latch or transfer colostrum at that time, it may be beneficial to have the mother pump her breasts immediately following the infant's initial attempts at feeding. Mothers should obtain and use a high quality hospital grade breast pump and express milk after each breastfeeding attempt and/or 8-10 times each 24 hours for the first 2 weeks or until the baby is established at the breast. Most mothers will need to pump until the infant reaches 40-42 weeks post menstrual age, as preterm infants usually do not drain the breasts well enough for the mother to stop pumping until the infant's due date has been reached. Mothers should wean from pumping by dropping one pumping per day per week until she either discontinues or pumps 1-2 times for storage (if returning to work).

FITTING THE FLANGE

The nurse or lactation consultant should help the mother select a properly fitting flange or breast shield. As nipples swell during pumping, it is important that the nipple be able to move freely once it is drawn into the shield's tunnel (Wilson-Clay & Hoover, 2002). If the nipple becomes strangulated in the shield's tunnel, soreness, reduced milk flow, and low milk supply can result. Standard pump kits provide flanges whose nipple tunnel opening is 24 mm to 25 mm, but many mothers benefit from a larger opening of 27 mm to 30 mm, which avoids nipple pain and results in more effective pumping (Meier et al., 2004).

OPTIMIZING MILK PRODUCTION

Following discharge, mothers can use cluster or power pumping several times a day to increase milk output if needed. This involves pumping for about 10 minutes or so or until as much milk as possible has been released from the first let down, then pumping again 10 to 20 minutes later to "trick" the breasts into another "first" letdown. The first let down can produce almost half of the total volume of milk in the breast (Ramsay et al., 2006). Milk production should be watched very carefully during the first 14 days following delivery, as there is a high potential for insufficient milk (Hill et al., 2005). Mothers who are exclusively or predominantly pumping should target a minimal output of 3500 ml/week (500 ml/day) by the end of the second week to achieve optimal output for sustained lactation (Hill et al., 1999). The optimal volume of milk by 10-14 days postpartum is >750 ml/24 hours, with outputs of <350 ml/24 hours placing the milk supply at an extremely high risk of remaining insufficient (Hurst & Meier, 2005). Milk volumes that reach 800-1000 ml/24 hours by 10-14 days provides a reserve such that if the maternal milk supply drops by as much as 50% during the infant's hospitalization, sufficient volume will remain to adequately nourish her infant upon discharge from the hospital (Hurst & Meier, 2005). Mothers of twins should target a minimum of 1000 ml/24 hours of pumped milk, assuming that 500 ml/day is the minimum for singleton infants.

PUTTING IT ALL TOGETHER

The birth of a late preterm infant can be emotionally grueling on new parents, especially when a deceptively healthy-looking infant is subjected to high-risk interventions. Breastfeeding success will improve if the maternity unit utilizes an evidence-based protocol (Table 4).

To assure consistent and effective care, the nurse, lactation consultant, and mother should mutually construct written feeding plans for use in the hospital and following discharge (Wight, 2003). With twins or higher order multiples, different feeding plans may need to be created for each infant. Mothers should have an appointment with the baby's primary care provider within 2 days of discharge if leaving the hospital within 72 hours. Another visit may be warranted at 5 to 7 days of age when bilirubin levels are likely to peak.

Preterm infants should be positioned so that their head, neck, and trunk are in straight alignment. They should not be in extreme flexion (crumpled over). Car seats and slings can be a problem for the late preterm infant. Respiratory instability in the upright, scrunched position is a common problem with preterm infants (Merchant et al., 2001). Decreased muscle tone in the oropharynx, neck, and chest can result in compromise of the airway when the infant sits in an upright, scrunched position. The infant's safety in a car seat should be ascertained prior to discharge. Parents need to be advised that their baby may have a decreased tolerance for sitting for long periods of time in a car seat. Also, in regards to safety in confined positions, parents should be cautioned about the use of baby slings for the late preterm infant. While slings are a wonderful mechanism for keeping baby close and for breastfeeding and soothing needs, the flexed position in a sling may not be appropriate until the baby is a little older. Mothers need to use slings that can accommodate a small infant in an upright position or may find that baby wraps work better in avoiding extreme flexion (Walker, 2008). Mothers should be given written information on the care of the late preterm infant, as well as the name and contact information for a lactation consultant with the IBCLC credential for breastfeeding follow-up (Table 9).

Table 9. Resources for Parents of Late Preterm Infants

Title of Publication	Available from	Comments
Parent Guide: Going home with your late preterm infant	Contemporary Pediatrics *http://www.modernmedicine. com/modernmedicine/ Parent+Guides/Parent-Guide-Going-home-with-your-late-preterm-inf/ ArticleStandard/Article/deta il/473739?contextCategory Id=6465*	Accessed August 29, 2008
Late Preterm (Near-Term Infant: What Parents Need to Know	AWHONN *http://www.awhonn. org/awhonn/content. do?name=02_ PracticeResources/2C3_ Focus_NearTermInfant.htm*	Accessed August 29, 2008
Newborn Jaundice	Stokowski, L.A. 2002. Newborn jaundice. Advances in Neonatal Care, 2, 115.	

Title of Publication	Available from	Comments
ILCA's Inside Track: Breastfeeding Your Baby Who Arrived Slightly Early	http://www.ilca.org/ membership/JHL// nov07/07NovemberITBW. pdf (members only)	ILCA. 2007. Breastfeeding your baby who arrived slightly early. Journal of Human Lactation, 23, 269-270.
The Diaper Diary (for keeping track of output) and Pumping Milk for Your Premature Baby	http://www.lactnews.com/ ddiary.html	Accessed August 29, 2008
Breastfeeding with the supplementary nursing system	www.breastfeeding-support.de	Guoth-Gumberger M. 2006. Breastfeeding with the supplementary nursing system. Rosenheim, Germany
Name and contact information of a lactation consultant with the IBCLC credential	www.ilca.org/falc.html	Accessed August 29, 2008
Massachusetts Breastfeeding Coalition Zip Milk - to locate lactation consultants and other sources of breastfeeding support in Massachusetts	www.massbfc.org	Accessed August 29, 2008

Feeding Plans Following Discharge

Clinicians and mothers find it beneficial to mutually create an individualized breastfeeding plan for use following discharge. A sample plan appears below (Table 10). It can and should be modified to best provide mothers with the tools they need to successfully breastfeed their infants.

Table 10. Sample Plan for Breastfeeding Your Late Preterm Infant

Breastfeeding and your milk are very important to your late preterm baby. Even though your baby may look full-term, he/she is not fully developed and may need some extra help learning to breastfeed. Your milk contains ingredients that provide protection from disease and help promote your baby's brain development that was interrupted by an early birth. Your baby may tire easily before a feeding is finished and may seem to sleep a lot. These guidelines will help get breastfeeding off to a good start.
Feed your baby on cue 8-12 times each 24 hours. Early babies are not always reliable in telling you when they need to feed. Sleeping is not an indication that baby is getting enough. Use the following cues to tell you when to start a feeding, as this is when he is ready and available: • Rapid eye movements under the eyelids • Sucking movements of the mouth and tongue • Hand-to-mouth movements • Body movements • Small sounds (crying is a late sign of hunger and baby may not feed well)
Place your baby in a clutch or cross cradle position.
As your baby latches on, make sure his mouth is wide open.
You should hear or feel your baby swallowing every 1-3 sucks during most of the feeding.
Use alternate massage on each breast at each feeding to keep baby sucking and increase the amount of milk he receives at each feeding. Thoroughly massage and compress each part of the breast so that milk does not back up and set the stage for an infection.
If you are not sure how much milk he is getting at each feeding, you can weigh baby before and after a feeding. This will help you know if you need to offer a supplement.

Record each feeding, whether a supplement is used, the amount of pumped milk, the number of wet diapers, and the number of bowel movements on your feeding log until baby is reliably feeding and gaining weight.

If your baby does not latch to the breast, try the following:

- Gently roll your nipple between your fingers to make it easier for the baby to grasp.

- As you bring your baby to breast, have a helper place a tube feeding device or dropper in the corner of the baby's mouth and deliver a small amount of milk as the baby attempts to latch. If the baby swallows and attempts to latch again, another small amount of milk can be given. Repeat until baby no longer attempts to latch. These practice sessions should not last longer than 10 minutes to avoid tiring both you and your baby.

- Finish the feeding by finger or cup feeding.

- If the attempts at latching do not work, you may find that a silicone nipple shield will allow the baby to latch and sustain sucking at the breast. Moisten the shield with warm water, turn almost inside-out as you apply it to the breast, apply a little breastmilk to the outside of the shield, hand express milk into the shield tunnel, and bring the baby to breast. If the baby latches, continue using alternate massage throughout the feeding.

Baby should have at least 6 wet diapers and 3 or more bowel movements each day by the 5th day. Bowel movements should start turning yellow by day 4. Meconium diapers on day 5 may indicate that baby is not getting enough milk. Uric acid crystals (red stains) on day 4 in wet diapers may also indicate that baby is not transferring enough milk at the breast.

Take your baby to his physician's office 2 days after coming home from the hospital for a weight check and to make sure he is not jaundiced. A weight check every 3 days or so assures that your baby continues to gain about 1/2 to 1 ounce per day.

If baby cannot feed long enough at each feeding or is not gaining well, supplements of expressed breastmilk can be given by tube feeding at the breast, finger feeding, cup feeding, or bottle feeding. If you do not have enough milk to use as a supplement, a hydrolyzed formula can be used until your milk production has increased.

Continue to pump your milk 2 to 3 times each day to use as a supplement and to improve your milk supply. Try "power pumping" once or twice each day. Pump for 5 to 10 minutes until the milk stops spraying from the first let down. Wait 15 to 20 minutes and pump again until the milk stops spraying. Almost half of the milk that is available in the breast is pumped with the first let down. Power pumping takes advantage of these "first" letdowns to mimic frequent feedings and helps increase your milk production. Depending on how your baby is doing at the breast, pumping should continue until he is 40-42 weeks corrected age, weaning off the pump over the first month home.

Conclusion

Assisting the mother of a late preterm infant learn how best to breastfeed her infant can be time consuming and frustrating. It will call upon the clinician's diagnostic and assessment skills and knowledge base of breastfeeding in special situations. The health benefits of breastfeeding and/or the provision of mother's own milk until the infant is established at the breast validate the increased use of health provider time to see that this happens. Because it is an investment in health that lasts a lifetime, it is worth the time, effort, and patience!

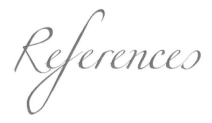

References

Academy of Breastfeeding Medicine. (2006). ABM Clinical Protocol #1: Guidelines for glucose monitoring and treatment of hypoglycemia in breastfed neonates. Revision June 2006. Retrieved August 29, 2008, from http://www.bfmed.org/ace-files/protocol/hypoglycemia.pdf.

Adamkin, D.H. (2006). Feeding problems in the late preterm infant. Clinics in Perinatology, 33, 831-837.American Academy of Pediatrics (AAP) Subcommittee on Hyperbilirubinemia. (2004). Management of hyperbilirubinemia in the newborn infant 35 or more weeks of gestation. Pediatrics, 114, 297–316.

Arthur, P.G., Smith, M., & Hartmann, P.E. (1989). Milk lactose, citrate, and glucose as markers of lactogenesis in normal and diabetic women. Journal of Pediatric Gastroenterology and Nutrition, 9, 488-496.

Askin, D.F., Bakewell-Sachs, S., Medoff-Cooper, B., Rosenberg, S., & Santa-Donato, A. (2008). Late preterm infant assessment guide. Washington, DC: Association of Women's Health, Obstetric and Neonatal Nurses.

Aylward, G.P. (2005). Neurodevelopmental outcomes of infants born prematurely. Journal of Developmental and Behavioral Pediatrics, 26, 427-440.

Bader, A., Fragneto, R., Terui, K., Arthur, G., Lofeski, B., & Data, S. (1995). Maternal and neonatal fentanyl and bupivacaine concentrations after epidural infusion during labor. Anesthesia and Analgesia, 81, 829-832.

Bakr, A.F., Abbas, M.M. (2006). Severe respiratory distress in term infants born electively at high altitude. BMC Pregnancy Childbirth, 6, 4.

Bekkali, N., Hamers, S.L., Schipperus, M.R., Reitsma, J.B., Valerio, P.G., Van Toledo, L., & Benninga, M.A. (2008). Duration of meconium passage in preterm and term infants. Archives of Diseases in Childhood, 93, F376-F379.

Beilin, Y., Bodian, C.A., Weiser, J., Hossain, S., Arnold, I., Feierman, D.E., Martin, G., & Holzman, I. (2005) Effect of labor epidural analgesia with and without fentanyl on infant breast-feeding: a prospective, randomized, double-blind study. Anesthesiology, 103, 1211-1217.

Bergman, N.J., Linley, L., & Fawcus, S.R. (2004). Randomized controlled trial of skin-to-skin contact from birth versus conventional incubator for physiological stabilization in 1200- to 2199-gram newborns. Acta Paediatrica, 93, 779-785.

Bettegowda, V.R., Dias, T., Davidoff, M.J., Damus, K., Callaghan W.M., & Petrini, J.R. (2008). The relationship between cesarean delivery and gestational age among US singleton births. Clinics in Perinatology, 35, 309-323.

Bettes, B.A., Coleman, V.H., Zinberg, S., Spong, C.Y., Portnoy, B., DeVoto, E., & Schulkin, J. (2007). Cesarean delivery on maternal request: obstetrician-gynecologists' knowledge, perception, and practice patterns. Obstetrics and Gynecology, 109, 57-66.

Bhutani, V.K. & Johnson, L. (2006). Kernicterus in late preterm infants cared for as term healthy infants. Seminars in Perinatology, 30, 89-97.

Bhutani, V.K., Johnson, L., & Sivieri, E.M. (1999). Predictive ability of a predischarge hour-specific serum bilirubin for subsequent significant hyperbilirubinemia in healthy term and near-term newborns. Pediatrics, 103, 6–14.

Boucher, N., Bairam, A., & Beaulac-Baillargeon, L. (2008). A new look at the neonate's clinical presentation after in utero exposure to antidepressants in late pregnancy. Journal of Clinical Psychopharmacology, 28, 334-339.

Bromiker, R., Rachamim, A., Hammerman, C., Schimmel, M., Kaplan, M., & Medoff-Cooper, B. (2006). Immature sucking patterns in infants of mothers with diabetes. The Journal of Pediatrics, 149, 640-643.

Bystrova, K., Widstrom, A.M., Matthiesen, A.S., Ransjo-Arvidson, A.B., Welles-Nystrom, B., Wassberg, C., et al. (2003). Skin-to-skin contact may reduce negative consequences of "the stress of being born": a study on temperature in newborn infants subjected to different ward routines in St. Petersburg. Acta Paediatrica, 92, 320-326.

Chapman, D.J. & Perez-Escamilla, R. (1999). Identification of risk factors for delayed onset of lactation. Journal of the American Dietetic Association, 99, 450-454.

Chertok, I.R., Schneider, J., & Blackburn, S. (2006). A pilot study of maternal and term infant outcomes associated with ultrathin nipple shield use. Journal of Obstetric, Gynecologic, and Neonatal Nursing, 35, 265-272.

Christensson, K., Siles, C., Moreno, L., Belaustequi, A., De la Fuente, P., Lagercrantz, H., et al. (1992). Temperature, metabolic adaptation and crying in healthy, full-term newborns cared for skin-to-skin or in a cot. Acta Paediatrica, 81, 488-493.

Chyi, L.J., Lee, H.C., Hintz, S.R., Gould, J.B., & Sutcliffe, T.L. (2008). School outcomes of late preterm infants: special needs and challenges for infants born at 32 to 36 weeks gestation. The Journal of Pediatrics, 153, 25-31.

Clements, K.M., Barfield, W.D., Ayadi, M.F., & Wilber, N. (2007). Preterm birth-associated cost of early intervention services: An analysis by gestational age. Pediatrics, 119, e866-e874.

Colson, S.D., de Rooy, L., & Hawdon, J.M. (2003). Biological nurturing increases duration of breastfeeding for a vulnerable cohort. MIDIRS Midwifery Digest, 13, 92-97.

Cotterman, K.J. (2004). Reverse pressure softening: a simple tool to prepare areola for easier latching during engorgement. Journal of Human Lactation, 20, 227-237.

Cowan, W.M. (1979). The development of the brain. Scientific American, 241, 113-133.

Cox, S.G. (2006). Expressing and storing colostrum antenatally for use in the newborn period. Breastfeeding Review, 14, 11-16.

Cregan, M.D., De Mello, T.R., Kershaw, D., McDougall, K., & Hartmann, P.E. (2002). Initiation of lactation in women after preterm delivery. Acta Obstetrica Gynecologica Scandanavia, 81, 870-877.

Dabrowski, G.A. (2007). Skin-to-skin contact: giving birth back to mothers and babies. Nursing for Women's Health, 11, 66-71.

Danner, S.C. & Cerutti, E.R. (1984). Nursing your neurologically impaired baby. Rochester, NY: Childbirth Graphics.

Darnall, R.A., Ariagno, R.L., & Kinney, H.C. (2006). The late preterm infant and the control of breathing, sleep, and brainstem development: a review. Clinics in Perinatology, 33, 883-914.

Davidoff, M.J., Dias, T., Damus, K., Russell, R., Bettegowda, V.R., Dolan, S., et al. (2006). Changes in the gestational age distribution among U.S. singleton births: impact on rates of late preterm birth. Seminars in Perinatology, 30, 8-15.

Declercq, E.R., Sakala, C., Corry, M.P., Applebaum, S., & Risher, P. (2002). Listening to mothers: report of the first national U.S. survey of women's childbearing experiences. New York: Maternity Center Association.

Desprats, R., Dumas, J.C., Giroux, M., Campistron, G., Faure, F., Teixeira, M.G., et al. (1991). Maternal and umbilical cord concentrations of fentanyl after epidural analgesia for cesarean section. European Journal of Obstetrics, Gynecology, and Reproductive Biology, 42, 89-94.

Dewey, K.G. (2001). Maternal and fetal stress are associated with impaired lactogenesis in humans. The Journal of Nutrition, 131, 3012S-3015S.

Dewey, K.G., Nommsen-Rivers, L.A., Heinig, M.J., & Cohen, R.J. (2003). Risk factors for suboptimal infant breastfeeding behavior, delayed onset of lactation, and excess neonatal weight loss. Pediatrics, 112, 607-619.

Doumouchtsis, S.K. & Arulkumaran, S. (2008). Head trauma after instrumental births. Clinics in Perinatology, 35, 69-83.

Dowling, D.A., Meier, P.P., DiFiore, J.M., Blatz, M., & Martin, R.J. (2002). Cup-feeding for preterm infants: mechanics and safety. Journal of Human Lactation, 18, 13-20.

Edgehouse, L. & Radzyminski, S.G. (1990). A device for supplementing breastfeeding. American Journal of Maternal and Child Nursing, 15, 34-35.

Eliot, L. (1999). What's going on in there: how the brain and mind develop in the first five years of life. New York: Bantam Books.

Engle, W.A. & Kominiarek, M.A. (2008). Late preterm infants, early term infants, and timing of elective deliveries. Clinics in Perinatology, 35, 325-341.

Engle, W.A., Tomashek, K.M., Wallman, C., & Committee on Fetus and Newborn, American Academy of Pediatrics. (2007). "Late-preterm" infants: a population at risk. Pediatrics, 120, 1390-1401.

Evans, K.C., Evans, R.G., Royal, R., Esterman, A.J., & James S.L. (2003). Effect of caesarean section on breast milk transfer to the normal term infant over the first week of life. Archives of Disease in Childhood. Fetal and Neonatal Edition, 88, F380-F382.

Ezaki, S., Ito, T., Suzuki, K., & Tamura, M. (2008). Association between total antioxidant capacity in breast milk and postnatal age in days in premature infants. Journal of Clinical and Biochemical Nutrition, 42, 133-137.

Fadavi, S., Punwani, I.C., Jain, L., & Vidyasagar, D. (1997). Mechanics and energetics of nutritive sucking: a functional comparison of commercially available nipples. Journal of Pediatrics, 130, 740-745.

Ferrante, A., Silvestri, R., & Montinaro, C. (2006). The importance of choosing the right feeding aids to maintain breastfeeding after interruption. International Journal of Orofacial Myology, 32, 58-67.

Food and Drug Administration. (2005). Nubain. Retrieved April 17, 2008, from http:// www.fda.gov/medwatch/safety/2005/aug_PI/Nubain_PI.pdf.

Fuchs, K. & Wagner, R. (2006). Elective cesarean section and induction and their impact on late preterm births. Clinics in Perinatology, 33, 793-801.

Furman, L. & Minich, N.M. (2006). Evaluation of breastfeeding of very low birth weight infants. Can we use the Infant Breastfeeding Assessment Tool? Journal of Human Lactation, 22, 175-181.

Gartner, L.M. & Herschel, M. (2001). Jaundice and breastfeeding. Pediatric Clinics in North America, 48, 389-399.

Geddes, D.T., Kent, J.C., Mitoulas, R., & Hartmann, P.E. (2008). Tongue movement and intra-oral vacuum in breastfeeding infants. Early Human Development, 84, 471-477.

Genna, C.W., Fram, J.L., & Sandora, L. (2008). Neurological issues and breastfeeding. In C.W. Genna, Supporting sucking skills in breastfeeding infants. Sudbury, MA: Jones and Bartlett Publishers.

Georgieff, M.K. (2006). The effect of maternal diabetes during pregnancy on the neurodevelopment of offspring. Minnesota Medicine, 89, 44-47.

Goldfield, E.C., Richardson, M.J., Lee, K.G., & Margetts, S. (2006). Coordination of sucking, swallowing, and breathing and oxygen saturation during early infant breastfeeding and bottle-feeding. Pediatric Research, 60, 450-455.

Gomes, C.F., Trezza, E.M.C., Murade, E.C.M., & Padovani, C.R. (2006). Surface electromyography of facial muscles during natural and artificial feeding of infants. Journal of Pediatrics (Rio J), 82, 103-109.

Gourley, G.R., Li, Z., Kreamer, B.L., & Kosorok, M.R. (2005). A controlled, randomized, double-blind trial of prophylaxis against jaundice among breastfed newborns. Pediatrics, 116, 385-391.

Greer, F.R., Sicherer, S.H., Burks, A.W., American Academy of Pediatrics Committee on Nutrition, & American Academy of Pediatrics Section on Allergy and Immunology. (2008). Effects of early nutritional interventions on the development of atopic disease in infants and children: the role of maternal dietary restriction, breastfeeding, timing of introduction of complementary foods, and hydrolyzed formulas. Pediatrics, 121, 183-191.

Guoth-Gumberger, M. (2006). Breastfeeding with the supplementary nursing system. Rosenheim, Germany: Parent Info. Available from: www.breastfeeding-support.de.

Hake-Brooks, S.J. & Anderson, G.C. (2008). Kangaroo care and breastfeeding of mother-preterm infant dyads 0-18 months: a randomized, controlled trial. Neonatal Network, 27, 151-159.

Hale, T.W. (2008). Medications and mothers' milk. (13th Ed.). Amarillo, TX: Hale Publishing.

Hall, R.T., Mercer, A.M., Teasley, S.L., McPherson, D.M., Simon, S.D., Santos, S.R., et al. (2002). A breastfeeding assessment score to evaluate the risk for cessation of breastfeeding by 7 to 10 days of age. The Journal of Pediatrics, 141, 659-664.

Hamilton, B.E., Martin, J.A., & Ventura, S.J. (2007). Births: Preliminary data for 2006. National vital statistics reports; vol 56 no 7. Hyattsville, MD: National Center for Health Statistics.

Hamilton, B.E., Martin, J.A., & Ventura, S.J. (2006). Births: Preliminary data for 2005. Health-E-Stats. Released November 21, 2006.

Hankins, G.D.V., Clark, S., & Munn, M.B. (2006). Cesarean section on request at 39 weeks: impact on shoulder dystocia, fetal trauma, neonatal encephalopathy, and intrauterine fetal demise. Seminars in Perinatology, 30, 276-287.

Hartmann, P. & Cregan, M. (2001). Lactogenesis and the effects of insulin-dependent diabetes mellitus and prematurity. The Journal of Nutrition, 131, 3016S-3020S.

Hauth, J.C. (2006). Spontaneous preterm labor and premature rupture of membranes at late preterm gestations: to deliver or not to deliver. Seminars in Perinatology, 30, 98-102.

Heiskanen, N., Raatikainen, K., & Heinonen, S. (2006). Fetal macrosomia-a continuing obstetric challenge. Biology of the Neonate, 90, 98-103.

Helbo-Hansen, H. (1995). Neonatal effects of maternally administered fentanyl, alfentanil and sufentanil. In D. Bogod (Ed.), Balliere's clinical anesthesiology: obstetric anesthesia (pp. 675-689). London: Bailliere Tindall.

Hill, P.D., Aldag, J.C., & Chatterton, R.T. (1999). Effects of pumping style on milk production in mothers of non-nursing preterm infants. Journal of Human Lactation, 15, 209-216.

Hill, P.D., Aldag, J.C., & Chatterton, R.T. (2001). Initiation and frequency of pumping and milk production in mothers of non-nursing preterm infants. Journal of Human Lactation, 17, 9-11.

Hill, P.D., Aldag, J.C., Chatterton, R.T., & Zinaman, M. (2005). Comparison of milk output between mothers of preterm and term infants: the first 6 weeks after birth. Journal of Human Lactation, 21, 22-30.

Hillman, N. (2007). Hyperbilirubinemia in the late preterm infant. Newborn & Infant Nursing Reviews, 7, 91-94.

Hoover, K. (1998). Supplementation of the newborn by spoon in the first 24 hours. Journal of Human Lactation, 14, 245.

Howard, C.R., de Blieck, E.A., ten Hoopen, C.B., Howard, F.M., Lanphear, B.P., & Lawrence, R.A. (1999). Physiologic stability of newborns during cup- and bottle-feeding. Pediatrics, 104, 1204-1207.

Howard, C.R., Howard, F.M., Lanphear, B., Eberly, S., deBlieck, E.A., Oakes, D., & Lawrence, R.A. (2003). Randomized clinical trial of pacifier use and bottle-feeding or cup feeding and their effect on breastfeeding. Pediatrics, 111, 511-518.

Hurst, N. & Meier, P.P. (2005). Chaper 13: Breastfeeding the preterm infant. In: Riordan, J. (ed). Breastfeeding and human lactation. 3rd ed. Boston: Jones and Bartlett Publishers, p 376.

Hurst, N.M., Meier, P.P., & Engstrom, J.L. (1999). Mother's performing in-home measurement of milk intake during breastfeeding for their preterm infants: effects on breastfeeding outcomes at 1, 2, and 4 weeks post-NICU discharge. Pediatric Research, 45, 287A.

Hurst, N.M., Meier, P.P., Engstrom, J.L., & Myatt, A. (2004). Mothers performing in-home measurement of milk intake during breastfeeding of their preterm infants: maternal reactions and feeding outcomes. Journal of Human Lactation, 20, 178-187.

Hurst, N., Valentine, C.J., Renfro, L., Burns, P., & Ferlic, L. (1997). Skin-to-skin holding in the neonatal intensive care unit influences maternal milk volume. Journal of Perinatology, 17, 213-217.

Inoue, N., Sakashita, R., & Kamegai, T. (1995). Reduction of masseter muscle activity in bottle-fed babies. Early Human Development, 42, 185-193.

Jacobs, L.A., Dickinson, J.E., Hart, P.D., Doherty, D.A., & Faulkner, S.J. (2007). Normal nipple position in term infants measured on breastfeeding ultrasound. Journal of Human Lactation, 23, 52-59.

Jordan, S., Emery, S., Bradshaw, C., Watkins, A., & Friswell, W. (2005). The impact of intrapartum analgesia on infant feeding. BJOG: an International Journal of Obstetrics and Gynecology, 112, 927-934.

Karl, D.J. (2004). Using principles of newborn behavioral state organization to facilitate breastfeeding. American Journal of Maternal and Child Nursing, 29, 292-298.

Karlström, A., Engström-Olofsson, R., Norbergh, K.G., Sjöling, M., & Hildingsson, I. (2007). Postoperative pain after cesarean birth affects breastfeeding and infant care. Journal of Obstetric, Gynecologic, and Neonatal Nursing, 36, 430-440.

Kavanaugh, K., Mead, L., Meier, P., & Mangurten, H.H. (1995). Getting enough: mothers' concerns about breastfeeding a preterm infant after discharge. Journal of Obstetric, Gynecologic, and Neonatal Nursing, 24, 23-32.

Kent, J.C., Ramsay, D.T., Doherty, D., Larsson, M., & Hartmann, P.E. (2003). Response of breasts to different stimulation patterns of an electric breast pump. Journal of Human Lactation, 19, 179-187.

Kesaree, N., Banapurmath, C.R., Banapurmath, S., & Shamanur, K. (1993). Treatment of inverted nipples using a disposable syringe. Journal of Human Lactation, 9, 27-29.

King, J.C. (2006). Maternal obesity, metabolism, and pregnancy outcomes. Annual Review of Nutrition, 26, 271-291.

Kinney, H.C. (2006). The near-term (late preterm) human brain and risk for periventricular leukomalacia: a review. Seminars in Perinatology, 30, 81-88.

Koehntop, D.E., Rodman, J.H., Brundage, D.M., Hegland, M.G., & Buckley, J. J. (1986). Pharmacokinetics of fentanyl in neonates. Anesthesia and Analgesia, 65, 227-232.

Kramer, M.S., Demissie, K., Yang, H., Platt, R.W., Sauvé, R., & Liston, R. (2000). The contribution of mild and moderate preterm birth to infant mortality. Fetal and Infant Health Study Group of the Canadian Perinatal Surveillance System. The Journal of the American Medical Association, 284, 843-849.

Law-Morstatt, L., Judd, D.M., Snyder, P., Baier, R.J., & Dhanireddy, R. (2003). Pacing as a treatment technique for transitional sucking patterns. Journal of Perinatology, 23, 483-488.

Levinson-Castiel, R., Merlob, P., Linder, N., Sirota, L., & Klinger, G. (2006). Neonatal abstinence syndrome after in utero exposure to selective serotonin reuptake inhibitors in term infants. Archives of Pediatrics & Adolescent Medicine, 160, 173-176.

Loftus, J.R., Hill, H., & Cohen, S.E. (1995). Placental transfer and neonatal effects of epidural sufentanil and fentanyl administered with bupivacaine during labor. Anesthesiology, 83, 300-308.

Lothian, J.A. (1995). It takes two to breastfeed: the baby's role in successful breastfeeding. Journal of Nurse Midwifery, 40, 328-334.

Ludwig, S.M. (2007). Oral feeding and the late preterm infant. Newborn & Infant Nursing Reviews, 7, 72-75.

Maisels, M.J. & Kring, E.A. (1998). Length of stay, jaundice, and hospital readmission. Pediatrics, 101, 995-998.

Maisels, M.J. & Kring, E. (2006). Transcutaneous bilirubin levels in the first 96 hours in a normal newborn population of >35 weeks gestation. Pediatrics, 117, 1169-1173.

Malloy, M.H. & Freeman, D.H. Jr. (2000). Birth weight and gestational age-specific sudden infant death syndrome mortality: United States, 1991 versus 1995. Pediatrics, 105, 1227-1231.

March of Dimes. (2006). Late preterm birth: every week matters. Medical Perspectives on Prematurity. Available from: http://www.marchofdimes.com/files/MP_Late_Preterm_Birth-Every_Week_Matters_3-24-06.pdf.

Marinelli, K.A., Burke, G.S., & Dodd, V.L. (2001). A comparison of the safety of cup feedings and bottle feedings in premature infants whose mothers intend to breastfeed. Journal of Perinatology, 21, 350-355.

Martin, J.A., Hamilton, B.E., Sutton, P.D., Ventura, S.J. Menacker, F., Kirmeyer, S., et al. (2007). Births: final data for 2005. National Vital Statistics Reports, 56, 1-104.

Matthiesen, A.S., Ransjö-Arvidson, A.B., Nissen, E., & Uvnäs-Moberg, K. (2001). Postpartum maternal oxytocin release by newborns: effects of infant hand massage and sucking. Birth, 28, 13-19.

Meier, P.P., Brown, L.P., Hurst, N.M., Spatz, D.L., Engstrom, J.L., Borucki, L.C., & Krouse, A.M. (2000). Nipple shields for preterm infants: effect on milk transfer and duration of breastfeeding. Journal of Human Lactation, 16, 106-114.

Meier, P.P., Furman, L.M., & Degenhardt, M. (2007). Increased lactation risk for late preterm infants and mothers: evidence and management strategies to protect breastfeeding. Journal of Midwifery and Women's Health, 52, 579-587.

Meier, P.P., Motykowski, Y., & Zuleger, J.L. (2004). Choosing a correctly-fitted breastshield for milk expression. Medela Messenger, 21, 8-9.

Meier, P. & Pugh, E.J. (1985). Breastfeeding behavior of small preterm infants. The American Journal of Maternal Child Nursing, 10, 396-401.

Menacker, F., Declercq, E., & Macdorman, M.F. (2006). Cesarean delivery: background, trends, and epidemiology. Seminars in Perinatology, 30, 235-241.

Merchant, J. R., Worwa, C., Porter, S., Coleman, J.M., & deRegnier, R.A. (2001). Respiratory instability of term and near-term healthy newborn infants in car safety seats. Pediatrics, 108, 647-652.

Miller, V. & Riordan, J. (2004). Treating postpartum breast edema with areolar compression. Journal of Human Lactation, 20, 223-226.

Mizuno, K. & Ueda, A. (2006). Changes in sucking performance from nonnutritive sucking to nutritive sucking during breast and bottle-feeding. Pediatric Research, 59, 728-731.

Moore, E.R., Anderson, G.C., & Bergman, N. (2007). Early skin-to-skin contact for mothers and their healthy newborn infants. Cochrane Database of Systematic Reviews, Jul 18, (3):CD003519.

Morrison, B., Ludington-Hoe, S., & Anderson, G.C. (2006). Interruptions to breastfeeding dyads on postpartum day 1 in a university hospital. Journal of Obstetric, Gynecologic, & Neonatal Nursing, 35, 709–716.

Neubauer, S.H., Ferris, A.M., Chase, C.G., Fanelli, J., Thompson, C.A., Lammi-Keefe, C.J., et al. (1993). Delayed lactogenesis in women with insulin-dependent diabetes mellitus. The American Journal of Clinical Nutrition, 58, 54-60.

Newman, T.B., Liljestrand, P., & Escobar, G.J. (2005). Combining clinical risk factors with bilirubin levels to predict hyperbilirubinemia in newborns. Archives of Pediatrics and Adolescent Medicine, 159, 113-119.

Newton, M. & Newton, N.R. (1948). The let-down reflex in human lactation. Pediatrics, 33, 698-704.

NIH State-of-the-Science Conference Statement on cesarean delivery on maternal request. (2006). NIH Consensus and State-of-the-Science Statements, 23, 1-29.

Nissen, E., Uvnäs-Moberg, K., Svensson, K., Stock, S., Widström, A.M., & Winberg, J. (1996). Different patterns of oxytocin, prolactin but not cortisol release during breastfeeding in women delivered by caesarean section or by the vaginal route. Early Human Development, 45, 103-118.

Nordeng, H. & Spigset, O. (2005). Treatment with selective serotonin reuptake inhibitors in the third trimester of pregnancy: effects on the infant. Drug Safety, 28, 565-81.

Nyqvist, K.H. (2008). Early attainment of breastfeeding competence in very preterm infants. Acta Paediatrica, 97, 776-781.

Nyqvist, K.H., Färnstrand, C., Eeg-Olofsson, K.E., & Ewald, U. (2001). Early oral behaviour in preterm infants during breastfeeding: an electromyographic study. Acta Paediatrica, 90, 658-663.

Nyqvist, K.H., Rubertsson, C., Ewald, U., Sjödén, P.O. (1996). Development of the preterm infant breastfeeding behavior scale (PIBBS): a study of nurse-mother agreement. Journal of Human Lactation, 12, 207-219.

O'Hana, H.P., Levy, A., Rozen, A., Greemberg, L., Shapira, Y., & Sheiner, E. (2008). The effect of epidural analgesia on labor progress and outcome in nulliparous women. The Journal of Maternal, Fetal & Neonatal Medicine, 15, 1-5.

Ornoy, A., Ratzon, N., Greenbaum, C., Wolf, A., & Dulitzky, M. (2001). School-age children born to diabetic mothers and to mothers with gestational diabetes exhibit a high rate of inattention and fine and gross motor impairment. Journal of Pediatric Endocrinology & Metabolism, 14, 681-689.

Pados, B.F. (2007). Safe transition to home: preparing the near-term infant for discharge. Newborn & Infant Nursing Reviews, 7, 106-113.

Palmer, M.M. (1993). Identification and management of the transitional suck pattern in premature infants. Journal of Perinatal and Neonatal Nursing, 7, 66-75.

Peterson, B.S., Anderson, A.W., Ehrenkranz, R., Staib, L.H., Tageldin, M., Colson, E., et al. (2003). Regional brain volumes and their later neurodevelopmental correlates in term and preterm infants. Pediatrics, 111, 939-948.

Peterson, B.S., Vohr, B., Staib, L.H., Cannistraci, C.J., Dolberg, A., Schneider, K.C., et al. (2000). Regional brain volume abnormalities and long-term cognitive outcome in preterm infants. The Journal of the American Medical Association, 284, 1939-1947.

Pressler, J.L., Hepworth, J.T., LaMontagne, L.L., Sevcik, R.H., & Hesselink, L.F. (1999). Behavioral responses of newborns of insulin-dependent and nondiabetic, healthy mothers. Clinical Nursing Research, 8, 103-118.

Raju, T.N. (2008). Late-preterm births: challenges and opportunities. Pediatrics, 121, 402-403.

Raju, T.N., Higgins, R.D., Stark, A.R., & Leveno, K.J. (2006). Optimizing care and outcome for late-preterm (near-term) infants: a summary of the workshop sponsored by the National Institute of Child Health and Human Development. Pediatrics, 118, 1207-1214.

Ramsay, D.T., Kent, J.C., Owens, R.A., & Hartmann, P.E. (2004). Ultrasound imaging of milk ejection in the breast of lactating women. Pediatrics, 113, 361-367.

Ramsay, D.T., Mitoulas, L.R., Kent, J.C., Cregan, M.D., Doherty, D.A., Larsson, M. & Hartmann, P.E. (2006). Milk flow rates can be used to identify and investigate milk ejection in women expressing breast milk using an electric breast pump. Breastfeeding Medicine, 1, 14-23.

Rasmussen, K.M. & Kjolhede, C.L. (2004). Prepregnant overweight and obesity diminish the prolactin response to suckling in the first week postpartum. Pediatrics, 113, e465-e471.

Rizzo, T., Freinkel, N., Metzger, B.E., Hatcher, R., Burns, W.J., & Barglow, P. (1990). Correlations between antepartum maternal metabolism and newborn behavior. American Journal of Obstetrics and Gynecology, 163, 1458-1464.

Sarici, S.U., Serdar, M.A., Korkmaz, A., Erdem, G., Oran, O., Tekinalp, G., et al. (2004). Incidence, course, and prediction of hyperbilirubinemia in near-term and term newborns. Pediatrics, 113, 775-780.

Schytt, E., Lindmark, G., & Waldenström, U. (2005). Physical symptoms after childbirth: prevalence and associations with self-rated health. BJOG: An International Journal of Obstetrics and Gynaecology, 112, 210-217.

Shulte, F.J., Michaelis, R., Nolte, R., Albert, G., Parl, U., & Lasson, U. (1969). Brain and behavioural maturation in newborn infants of diabetic mothers. Part 1: Nerve conduction and EEG patterns. Neuropädiatrie, 1, 24-35.

Shapiro-Mendoza, C.K., Tomashek, K.M., Kotelchuck, M., Barfield, W., Nannini, A., Weiss, J., et al. (2008). Effect of late-preterm birth and maternal medical conditions on newborn morbidity risk. Pediatrics, 121, e223-e232.

Simonson, C., Barlow, P., Dehennin, N., Sphel, M., Toppet, V., Murillo, D., et al. (2007). Neonatal complications of vacuum-assisted delivery. Obstetrics and Gynecology, 109, 626-633.

Steer, P., Biddle, C., Marley, W., Lantz, R., & Sulik, P. (1992). Concentration of fentanyl in colostrum after an analgesic dose. Canadian Journal of Anaesthesia, 39, 231-235.

Stellwagen, L.M., Hubbard, E.T., & Wolf, A. (2007). The late preterm infant: a little baby with big needs. Contemporary Pediatrics, November 1.

Stephenson, T., Budge, H., Mostyn, A., Pearce, S., Webb, R., & Symonds, M.E. (2001). Fetal and neonatal adipose tissue maturation: a primary site of cytokine and cytokine-receptor action. Biochemical Society Transactions, 29, 80-85.

Sullivan, M.C. & Margaret, M.M. (2003). Perinatal morbidity, mild motor delay, and later school outcomes. Developmental Medicine & Child Neurology, 45, 104-112.

Symonds, M.E., Mostyn, A., Pearce, S., Budge, H., & Stephenson, T. (2003). Endocrine and nutritional regulation of fetal adipose tissue development. The Journal of Endocrinology, 179, 293-299.

Thorley, V. (1997). Cup feeding: problems created by incorrect use. Journal of Human Lactation, 13, 54-55.

Tita, A., Mercer, B., & Ramin, S. (2008). Abstract 86. Elective cesarean delivery before 39 weeks affects outcome. Society for Maternal-Fetal Medicine 28th Annual Meeting. Presented February 2, 2008.

Tomashek, K.M., Shapiro-Mendoza, C.K, Weiss, J., Kotelchuck, M., Barfield, W., Evans, S., et al. (2006). Early discharge among late preterm and term newborns and risk of neonatal morbidity. Seminars in Perinatology, 30, 61-68.

Vaarala, O., Knip, M., Paronen, J., Hämäläinen, A.M., Muona, P., Väätäinen, M., et al. (1999). Cow's milk formula feeding induces primary immunization to insulin in infants at genetic risk for type 1 diabetes. Diabetes, 48, 1389-1394.

Vahratian, A. (2008). Prevalence of overweight and obesity among women of childbearing age: results from the 2002 National Survey of Family Growth. Maternal and Child Health Journal, Apr 16, [Epub ahead of print].

Van den berg, K.A. (1990). Nippling management of the sick neonate in the NICU: the disorganized feeder. Neonatal Network, 9, 9-16.

Vohr, B.R., Poindexter, B.B., & Dusick, A.M. (2006). Beneficial effects of breast milk in the neonatal intensive care unit on the developmental outcome of extremely low birth weight infants at 18 months of age. Pediatrics, 118, e115-123.

Walker, M. (2008). Breastfeeding the late preterm infant. Journal of Obstetric, Gynecologic, and Neonatal Nursing, 37, 692-701.

Wang, M.L., Dorer, D.J., Fleming, M.P., & Catlin, E. (2004). Clinical outcomes of near-term infants. Pediatrics, 114, 372-376.

Wang, B., McVeagh, P., Petocz, P., & Brand-Miller, J. (2003). Brain ganglioside and glycoprotein sialic acid in breastfed compared with formula-fed infants. The American Journal of Clinical Nutrition, 78, 1024-1029.

Ward Platt, M. & Deshpande, S. (2005). Metabolic adaptation at birth. Seminars in Fetal & Neonatal Medicine, 10, 341-350.

Watchko, J.F. (2006). Hyperbilirubinemia and bilirubin toxicity in the late preterm infant. Clinics in Perinatology, 33, 839-852.

Wight, N.E. (2003). Breastfeeding the borderline (near-term) preterm infant. Pediatric Annals, 32, 329-36.

Wiklund, I., Edman, G., & Andolf, E. (2007). Cesarean section on maternal request: reasons for the request, self-estimated health, expectations, experience of birth and signs of depression among first-time mothers. Acta Obstetricia Gynecologica Scandinavica, 86, 451-456.

Wilson-Clay, B. & Hoover, K. (2002). The breastfeeding atlas. Austin, TX: LactNews Press.

Wolf, L.S. & Glass, R.P. (1992). Feeding and swallowing disorders in infancy. Tucson, AZ: Therapy Skill Builders.

Wolf , L.S. & Glass, R.P. (2008). The Goldilocks problem: milk flow that is not too fast, not too slow, but just right. In C.W. Genna, Supporting sucking skills in breastfeeding infants. Sudbury, MA: Jones and Bartlett Publishers.

Glossary

ALTERNATE MASSAGE/BREAST COMPRESSIONS - Mother massages and compresses breast each time baby pauses between sucking bursts. This reduces the effort needed by the baby to withdraw milk from the breast. All quadrants of each breast need to be massaged and compressed during each feeding to prevent milk stasis and lowered milk production from inadequate drainage.

APNEA - Brief pauses in breathing.

AREOLAR COMPRESSION/REVERSE PRESSURE SOFTENING - Mother presses fingers around areola to make indentations or pits that serve to expose the nipple, making it easier for baby to latch to an engorged areola.

BIOLOGICAL NURTURING - Mother holds late preterm infants so that the baby's chest, abdomen, and legs are closely flexed around her body and unrestricted access to the breast is offered. It has been proposed that the preterm infant can continue to be incubated or gestated in the mother's arms during the early days following a late preterm birth.

BRADYCARDIA - A slow heartbeat which results in the heart not being able to pump enough blood to provide oxygen to the body.

BROWN FAT - Fat in newborn mammals used to generate body heat.

BUCCINATOR MUSCLES - Thin, flat muscle forming the wall of the cheek.

CEPHALHEMATOMA - A blood cyst, tumor, or swelling of the scalp of a newborn due to seeping of blood beneath the skin, often resulting from birth trauma.

CUP FEEDING - Infant is fed using a medicine cup. The medicine cup with a small amount of milk is placed against the infant's lower lip. The cup is tipped so that the milk is available to the infant when his tongue protrudes. The infant slowly sips or laps the milk.

DANCER HAND POSITION - Mother supports baby's chin during breastfeeding so that baby does not slip off nipple or bite or clench jaws to keep from sliding off breast.

DIGITAL INFANT SCALE - Scale used to weigh infant before and after feeding to determine amount ingested during the feed.

EARLY TERM INFANT - Infant born between 37 0/7 weeks and 38 6/7 weeks.

FINGER FEEDING - Infant is fed using a tube taped or held to a feeder's finger. The feeder's finger is placed pad side up and the infant is encouraged to draw the finger into his mouth. A small amount of milk is delivered through the tube when the infant sucks.

HALF-LIFE - Time required for half of a dose of a drug to be metabolized or eliminated from the body.

HYPOGLYCEMIA - Low blood sugar.

HYPOTHERMIA - Low body temperature.

HYPOTONIA - Low muscle tone.

IATROGENIC PRETERM BIRTH - Elective delivery of preterm infants.

JAUNDICE - Condition that results when bilirubin levels increase in the blood, resulting in yellowish staining of the eyes and skin. Extremely high levels in an infant can cause neurologic damage and possibly death.

KERNICTERUS - Chronic and permanent clinical outcomes of bilirubin toxicity, including athetoid cerebral palsy, hearing loss, paralysis of upward gaze, dental dysplasia, and possibly intellectual handicaps.

LACTOSE - A disaccharide found in milk composed of glucose and galactose – milk sugar.

LATE PRETERM INFANT - Infant born between 34 0/7 weeks and 36 6/7 weeks.

MANDIBLE - Lower jaw

MASSETER MUSCLE - Muscle involved in chewing, biting, swallowing, and speech.

MORBIDITY – Illness

MORTALITY – Death

MUSCLES INVOLVED IN MOVING TONGUE:
- **STYLOGLOSSUS MUSCLES** - Small, short muscles located on each side of the tongue that

links the sides of the tongue to the base of the skull. Contraction of these two muscles pulls the tongue back and up.

- **PALATOGLOSSUS MUSCLES** - Muscles that originate from the soft palate and insert on each side of the tongue. These muscles work together to raise the back of the tongue.

- **GENIOGLOSSUS MUSCLES** - Flat, triangular muscles that originate from the inner surface of the front of the lower jaw and the hyoid bone and insert on each side of the tip of the tongue. When the two muscles contract at the same time, the tongue is protruded by its whole foundation being pulled forward.

- **HYOGLOSSUS MUSCLES** - Thin, flat strap of muscle located on each side of the tongue. It originates from the side of the hyoid bone in the throat and passes vertically inside the tongue. When the two hyoglossus muscles contract, they depress the tongue and turn the sides down.

The genioglossus, styloglossus, palatoglossus, and hyoglossus muscles work together to move the tongue.

MYELINATION - Coating of the branches of nerve cells with a fatty substance to keep ions from leaking out. This coating speeds transmission of electrical signals along a nerve fiber.

NECROTIZING ENTEROCOLITIS (NEC) - Medical condition primarily seen in premature infants. NEC involves infection and inflammation that causes destruction of the bowel or part of the bowel.

NIPPLE TUG - Gentle tug on the nipple (or can pull baby slightly away) while infant is latched on, causing baby to draw the nipple/areola farther back into his mouth to maintain latch.

NOMOGRAM - Graph that looks at the infant's gestational age, age in hours post birth, and bilirubin level to predict the likelihood of severe jaundice.

OLIGOSACCHARIDES - Carbohydrate molecule composed of 3-20 simple sugars (monosaccharides).

OROPHARYNX - The part of the throat at the back of the mouth. It includes the soft palate, the base of the tongue, and the tonsils.

PACED FEEDING - Bottle feeding where feeder regulates infant suck/swallow/pauses by removing the nipple from the infant's mouth after every 3 to 5 sucks, allowing a 3-5 second pause for breathing. The nipple rests on the midpoint of the infant's upper lip during the pause, allowing the infant to draw the nipple back into the mouth when ready to resume feeding. With late preterm infants, the bottle can be tipped downward to stop the flow of liquid into the baby's mouth, giving the infant time to swallow and breathe.

PERIVENTRICULAR LEUKOMALACIA (PVL) - Death of white matter of the brain due to softening of the brain tissue. This is caused by a lack of oxygen or blood flow to the periventricular area of the brain, by bleeding into the brain, or by a bacterial infection in mother or infant that triggers a cytokine response in the brain.

POST TERM INFANT - Infant born at 42 weeks or beyond.

POWER PUMPING - Method of pumping to increase milk supply. Mothers pump for 5-10 minutes or until milk stops spraying from first let down, then wait 15-20 minutes and pump again until milk stops spraying. Power pumping takes advantage of first letdowns to mimic frequent feeding and helps increase milk production.

PREEMIE ACT - Legislation passed in 2006 that mandates research expansion, better provider education and training, and a Surgeon General's conference to address the growing epidemic of preterm births.

RETINOPATHY OF PREMATURITY - Potentially blinding eye disorder that primarily affects premature infants weighing less than 2 3/4 pounds or born before 31 weeks of gestation.

SEPSIS - Over reaction by the body to an infection.

SIALIC ACID – A chemical component of a number of complex chemical structures in the human body. A disturbance in sialic acid metabolism may lead to a concentration of sialic acid in the blood, urine or solid tissue. This almost always leads to physical and mental deterioration.

SUBCUTANEOUS FAT - Fatty or adipose tissue that lies directly under the skin.

SUBLINGUAL PRESSURE - Mother slips index finger directly behind and under the tip of the chin where the tongue attaches, limiting downward movement of the jaw so that suction is not broken each time the jaw drops.

TEMPORALIS MUSCLE - Muscle responsible for raising the mandible.

TERM INFANT - Infant born between 39 0/7 and 41 6/7 weeks of gestation.

VISUOMOTOR INTEGRATIVE SKILLS - Vision and movement working together to produce actions. Some of the complications of premature birth affect development of visuomotor skills.

Index

A

Abnormal breathing 13, 48

Academic achievement 11

Airway instability 5

Alternate massage 24, 25, 32, 37, 46, 55, 56

Apnea 5, 6, 11, 13, 16, 26, 44, 45

Areolar compression 30

Areolar edema 29

Artificial nipples 40, 43, 44, 45

Attention-deficit hyperactivity disorder 11

B

Baby wraps 53

Behavioral issues 11

Behavior rating scale 12

Bilirubin 14, 15, 46, 47

Bilirubin encephalopathy 15

Biological nurturing 23

Birth intervention 15

Bottles 40, 42

Bradycardia 5, 6, 13, 16, 26, 41, 44, 45, 48

Brain weight 11

Breast compressions 32

Breastfeeding plan of care 15, 21

Breastfeeding protocols 22

Breastmilk 12, 14, 15, 18, 42, 56, 80

Breast shield 51

C

Car seat 52

Centrally mediated apnea 13

Cephalhematoma 17

Cesarean 3, 5, 7, 8, 14, 15, 16, 18, 23, 40

Chronic lung disease 12

Cluster or power pumping 52

Clutch 26, 27, 28, 38, 55

Colostrum 18, 19, 24, 25, 26, 29, 32, 34, 37, 38, 46, 51

Counter-regulatory efforts 14

Cow's milk based formula 12

Cross cradle 26, 27

Cup feeding 39, 40, 44, 56

D

Dancer hand position 29, 30

Dehydration 5, 15, 18

Diabetic mothers 14, 21, 37, 38

Digital infant scale 42

E

Early intervention services 6

Early term 3

Epidural analgesia 16, 17

Excessive sleepiness 5, 15

Executive function 11

Extreme flexion 26, 52, 53

F

Feeding cues 23, 24, 51
Fentanyl 16, 17
Finger feeding 39, 41 - 43, 56
Flange 51
Flat nipples 31
Free radicals 12
Frequent startling 13, 48

G

Glucose 12, 13, 14, 21, 25
Glycogen stores 9, 13, 14
Gyri 13

H

Half-life 16
Hand expression 51
Human milk 12, 37, 39
Hydrolyzed formula 38, 56
Hyperbilirubinemia 14, 15, 18, 46
Hypoglycemia 5, 6, 13, 14, 22 - 24, 37
Hypothermia 5, 13, 21
Hypotonia 16, 29

I

Iatrogenic preterm birth 9
Immature self regulation 5, 48
Inductions 7, 9
Intraventricular hemorrhage 12
IQ 11, 12

J

Jaundice 5, 6, 14, 15, 46, 53, 56

K

Ketogenic response 14

L

Lactogenesis II 5, 17
Lactose 12
Language 11
Latch assistance 29
Late preterm 1, 3, 4, 6 - 9, 11 - 19, 22, 24, 41, 42, 45, 46, 48, 51 - 53
Late preterm infant initiative 4

M

March of Dimes 4
Maternal obesity 7, 8
Meconium 14, 46, 56
Mental development index 12
Milk ejection reflex 16
Milk incentives 37, 44
Milk production 5, 17, 18, 32, 43 - 45, 52, 56
Milk stasis 32, 35
Milk supply 5, 17, 21, 42, 51, 52, 56
Milk transfer 5, 18 - 20, 32, 62, 66
Morbidity 1, 6, 11
Mortality 1, 2, 7
Motor/neurologic function 11
Muscle tone 9, 13, 16, 17, 19, 20, 26, 29, 48, 52
Myelin 9
Myelination 9, 10, 12

N

Nalbuphine 16

National Institutes of Health 4

Near term 1, 4

Necrotizing enterocolitis 12

Nipple shield 33, 46, 56

Nipple tug 32

Nomogram 15, 46, 47

Nubain 16

Nutritive sucking 15, 29, 33, 40

O

Obesity 5, 7, 8, 14

Overweight 5, 8, 14, 17, 18

P

Paced feeding 41

Periventricular leukomalacia 11

Positions 26, 28, 53

Post term 3

Pre- and post-feed weights 42, 46

PREEMIE ACT 5

Preterm Infant Breastfeeding
Behavior Scale 35, 36

Psychomotor Development Index 12

Pumping 5, 37, 51, 52, 54

R

Respiratory distress 3, 5, 6, 13

Retinopathy of prematurity 12

Reverse pressure softening 30

S

Sample plan 55

Selective serotonin reuptake inhibitors 17

Self regulate 13

Self regulation 5, 48

Sepsis 3, 4, 5, 6, 14

Sialic acid 12

Skin mottling 13, 48

Slings 52, 53

Soy formula 12

Spitting up 48

Sublingual pressure 29

Sucking 5, 15, 16, 19 - 21, 23 - 25, 29,
32 - 36

Sudden infant death syndrome 7, 13

Sulci 13

Supplementation 5, 37, 38, 40 - 42, 45

T

Tachycardia 48

Temperature instability 6, 13

Term 1, 3, 9, 11, 13, 15, 17 - 21, 23, 25,
40, 48, 51

U

Uridine diphosphate
glucuronyl transferase 14

V

Vacuum extraction 17

Visuomotor integrative skills 11

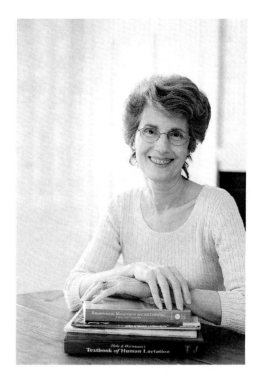

Meet the Author

Marsha Walker, RN, IBCLC is the Executive Director of the National Alliance for Breastfeeding Advocacy, Research, Education and Legal Branch (NABA REAL). She is a long time breastfeeding advocate, starting as a volunteer breastfeeding counselor with the Nursing Mothers Counsel in California. Marsha went on to become a childbirth educator through Lamaze International, a registered nurse, and an International Board Certified Lactation Consultant. She served on the Representative Panel of Experts in 1985, which constructed the first lactation consultant exam and was one of a number of clinicians on whose practice the exam grid is based. Marsha enjoyed a large clinical lactation practice at Harvard Pilgrim Health Plan, a major HMO in Massachusetts, where she was the Director of the Breastfeeding Support Program for 12 years. She has served on the Board of Directors of the International Lactation Consultant Association (ILCA) for 7 years, including as its president in 1999.

Marsha is on the Board of Directors of the Massachusetts Breastfeeding Coalition, Baby Friendly USA, and Best for Babes. She is ILCA's representative to the US Department of Agriculture's Breastfeeding Promotion Consortium and NABA's representative to the US Breastfeeding Committee. She has worked for 8 years to get breastfeeding legislation passed in her state of Massachusetts, which became a reality in January 2009. She is the co-chair of the Ban the Bags campaign, a national effort to eliminate the hospital distribution of formula company discharge bags.

NABA REAL is the IBFAN organization in the United States and is responsible for monitoring the International Code of Marketing of Breastmilk Substitutes in the US. Marsha has written both country reports on Code monitoring activities in the US, "Selling Out Mothers and Babies" and "Still Selling Out Mothers and Babies." Marsha is an international speaker on breastfeeding and an author of numerous publications, including her book "Breastfeeding Management for the Clinician: Using the Evidence."

Marsha is married and the mother of two breastfed children, Shannon (33) and Justin (32), her original breastfeeding clinical instructors. She is the grandmother of 4 breastfed girls - Haley, Sophie, Isabelle, and Ella.

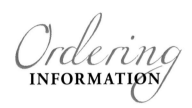

Ordering
INFORMATION

HALE PUBLISHING, L.P.

1712 N. Forest Street
Amarillo, Texas, USA 79106

❖

8:00 AM TO 5:00 PM CST

❖

CALL » 806.376.9900

SALES » 800.378.1317

FAX » 806.376.9901

❖

ONLINE WEB ORDERS
www.ibreastfeeding.com

❖